WHERE HAVE ALL THE STORKS GONE?

A HIS AND HERS GUIDE TO INFERTILITY

Michelle & Chris Miller

Family photographs by Melissa Glynn Photography
Book cover design by Henry Blas

www.wherehaveallthestorksgone.com

This book is dedicated to our friends and family. Their unwavering support inspired, and funded us, through the trials and tribulations of infertility.

Special thanks to Roger Porter, our awesome editor and good friend who helped us bring this book to life.

Contents

FOREWORD

I've seen countless couples like Michelle and Chris in my 33 years as a fertility subspecialist. But, I've never had a couple share their life story with me (at least, not in book form). When they asked me to write this foreword, I wasn't sure where to begin. And then I thought about the journey they shared with me and knew exactly what to say.

As a physician, I evaluate and treat couples for infertility and conduct research. Some patients require surgery, some require medications and some require a combination of both to improve their fertility. But research shows that our emotions and attitudes profoundly affect our bodies and, therefore, affect the chance of success of fertility treatments. Michelle and Chris use their individual perspectives to give a full picture of infertility through their story—both the science and the heart.

So, read on and enjoy a romantic love story and a step-by-step guide to infertility all wrapped into one. Their words will encourage you—and those closest to you—to laugh, to cry, to share, and to support each other as you embark on your own journey.

DR. THOMAS C. VAUGHN

"Learn from yesterday, live for today, hope for tomorrow. The important thing is to not stop questioning."
— Albert Einstein

PROLOGUE

When the time comes to start a family, most couples don't expect to encounter difficulty conceiving. Why should we? We're warned at a young age that it only takes one mistake to get pregnant. We hear stories or see examples of unplanned conceptions all the time. Precisely what our friend's father alluded to with his warning the day his son started high school—"Don't paint yourself into a corner, Trey!"

What I never realized is that when we're ready and willing to paint ourselves into that corner, it doesn't always happen easily. We rarely hear stories of couples trying to conceive who are unsuccessful—until it happens to us. I always assumed that any couple without children had simply chosen that path. It never crossed my mind that they could have desperately wanted a child and had simply been denied by biology.

Infertility affects more than seven million couples in the United States and 80 million couples worldwide.

At one in six couples, the odds are that you or someone you know has had trouble conceiving.

What exactly is infertility? The label is typically placed on those who have been trying to conceive for at least one year without success. Conception depends on several factors. At the most basic level, it requires a healthy sperm, healthy egg, the means for both to join and fertilize into a quality embryo which implants successfully, as well as adequate hormone levels to sustain the pregnancy. A problem with any one of these factors can result in infertility.

This book was written for anyone interested in the topic of fertility. Those who are trying to conceive—whether you've just begun the process or you've struggled with infertility for years. Those who've already been through it all and want to look back and have a laugh. And maybe most of all, to serve as a guide for the families and friends of couples dealing with this issue. Even with the best intentions, your comments may be impolite, insensitive or hurtful, so our hope is that by reading this book, you can understand a little more and perhaps say a little less.

Our primary goal is to share a little humor and give you both a woman's perspective (noted by the Venus symbol ♀), and a man's perspective (noted by the Mars symbol ♂) in all things fertility. We'll also try to impart a little knowledge and some definitions along the way so you won't have to do a Google search after every paragraph. Any term or process underlined in this book is defined in more detail in Appendix A. If you do find yourself confused at any point, it's my husband, Chris' fault. The man's always to blame, isn't he?

I believe in fairy tales. I believe that wishes do come true (although sometimes that means a lot of hard work and a little luck). But wishes don't always come true precisely how you want or expect them to. That to me is the magic and irony of life.

The fertility process is confusing, frustrating, arduous, torturous and excruciating. Nothing can prepare you for it. It can linger like shadows and haunt you like a ghost. But hopefully, you will find a little magic in the process as well. My advice is—don't let it all get to you. And I know that's easier said than done.

This book won't answer all of your questions. It may not answer any of them. But I hope to share our experiences, my knowledge (however limited that may be) and in many cases, my opinions. I hope that somewhere in this book you find something that makes you laugh, helps you grow, or maybe best of all, helps you achieve your dreams—fertility or otherwise.

You are probably reading this because you are trying to conceive or someone close to you is going through the process. I set one main goal and that is to give you an honest and somewhat humorous glimpse into one couple's story.

No matter what path you take, it has been treaded before. Not just by Michelle and me but by millions of couples before us. Many of the stories in this book have been so generously shared by family, friends and acquaintances. We carry their tales, like tiny parchments in a pouch, drawing them out when we need help or encouragement.

Throughout our ordeal, we read fertility-related books, articles and blogs to try to find information on what we should expect. There were two very distinct things missing. First, I felt like the science and statistics were often lacking. I'd often find myself doing secondary searches on topics to better understand the odds or the process overall. Second, there is little humor on the topic. And if I ever needed a little humor, it was definitely during this process!

The fertility process is, in and of itself, not in any way funny. But as humans, we are so often in helpless positions. We are at the mercy of our bodies, of science and often our surroundings. So I feel if I can't laugh at myself in this situation, at this sometimes hopeless and often embarrassing process, then what can I laugh at? And since stress doesn't help your chances of success—stress, it turns out, can be your sole enemy—then I think this means laughter is our friend.

My wife will tell you a number of stories about me and I am sure that all of them are at least in part true.

The whole truth is that I am lucky to have her. Just ask any of my friends and they will tell you. So will her family—and mine for that matter. One of my mentors once told me it was quite likely the greatest sale I've ever closed. For my part, I know all of this and I will spend my entire life trying to earn her love.

What does this all have to do with infertility? Aside from the obvious background about us, it should also give you some idea about my goals and perspective. My goal is to entertain her and make sure that she is happy. This was true throughout our fertility saga but also in our life overall. So while it may seem that I am too cavalier, or over the top in my actions and words, my judge is always Michelle's true happiness.

You may also be thinking, 'What the heck can a man tell you about the infertility process?' The answer is, maybe nothing. After all, I will not be the one on the table when labor starts. Well actually, I have been on the table, but that is a story for later. I only hope I can be honest and share my feelings and observations. Through this process with Michelle, I have seen my clear and unaltered purpose was to make her laugh, keep her happy and often just to give her a shoulder to cry upon. You too will need to find your purpose, your balance and your own road.

PART I

WE HAVE LIFT-OFF

THE PROJECT BEGINS

The sun seems brighter today, I feel lighter and I'm radiating with joy. I am giddier than a toddler on Christmas morning. After nearly a year of begging, pleading, coaxing and bargaining, Chris has agreed to start trying for a baby.

My mother-in-law had come up with a crafty idea. She suggested that I stop taking birth control pills and then just act dumbfounded when the stick turned blue. She explained, "You know, you just can't wait around for the Miller boys. If I'd waited for Harold to say he was ready, we wouldn't have any children." When I laughed, a bit uncomfortably, she added with a stern, authoritative tone, "You think I'm kidding, but I am really serious." I certainly believe her, since their oldest daughter was born within a year of their marriage.

Chris and I have been married for a little less than three years, so most people would shrug their shoulders and ask, "What's the hurry?" Actually, until a year ago, I had rarely thought about having children—aside from knowing I probably wanted to at some point in my life. Then one day I was suddenly, inexplicably ready. Ready to be pregnant. And ready for all the responsibility that comes with it (I think!). And once you discover how long Chris and I dated and then add to that the three years of engagement, you'll know we've had ample time to prepare for this next step.

THE AGREEMENT

When Michelle approached me about wanting to get pregnant, I wasn't ready. Not because I don't want to have a child—I do, very much. I find kids much more entertaining than adults. And I love their honesty— that they say what's in their hearts.

But I am not naïve; I understand the magnitude of impact this will have on our lives and I have infinite respect for the responsibility of actually raising a child. If my parents taught me one thing, it was to have respect for responsibility. And I can't think of anything that will require more responsibility in my life than raising a son or daughter.

There is also the fact that, as a child, one of my most painful memories is of my parents' financial woes. Michelle and I have just begun to dig out of a gaping credit card sinkhole and that makes me nervous. I promised myself I would never put my child through that.

In all honesty, there are also the selfish reasons that I must mention. First, I love my wife and I really cherish the time I get to spend with her. We spend all the time we can together. I wake up early on weekends to ride my bike while she is still sleeping so I don't miss much time with her. I know that our alone time will be severely impacted by a new addition to the family.

Also, I am a 12-year-old at heart. I like being the youngest in the household. I love it when my wife spoils me rotten. You wouldn't believe the towering stacks of presents splayed in our living room on Christmas morning (recall the gaping credit card sinkhole). But even as I write these words, I realize that I will enjoy teaching my child about sharing and making sure that he or she is happy, even when it is at my expense.

So there you have it—the selfish and the fearful reasons that make me hesitate. But hesitations aside, I do want children and Michelle is very ready.

I agree to start trying.

I know what I am getting myself into. What could be tough to understand? It's lots of sex, followed by a ton of responsibility, right? I love sex, so at least that part should be a piece of cake.

LESSON 1: THINGS AREN'T ALWAYS
AS EASY AS THEY SEEM.

RELATIONSHIP TRENDS

All of the relationships I had before Chris never lasted very long. Take my first kiss. I was in the third grade and Doug, the cutest boy in our class (at least that's what I remember thinking at the time), was walking me home. When we were saying our goodbyes, he leaned in and gave me a gentle kiss. The electricity shot through the ends of my toes, lighting me up like a Christmas tree. In typical boy fashion, he slumped away and never mentioned it again.

This was huge news in a girl's life and it must have been written on my face because my big sister and her best friend clucked around like barnyard hens and pecked out my brains with jokes and giggles. I sat through an eternity of torture and mockery—or at least ten minutes worth—until finally, Jack, from *All*

My Children confessed to sleeping with his fiancé's sister who was supposed to be dead—and then the boisterous hens turned their eyes back to the television, distracted by more pressing issues. I survived my first girl talk.

My first crush was Chip, a confident, boisterous fifth grader with dark black hair and big brown eyes who was always laughing.

Starting a new relationship was so easy in those days. You tell your friend to tell his friend you like him. He tells his friend to tell your friend he likes you back. And then, eventually, you start talking without the help of your friends. My relationship with Chip never even got off the ground. Either my friend failed to communicate to his friend successfully or he wasn't interested.

I was in the eighth grade when I had my first official boyfriend. His name was Juan and he was trouble—the kind of boy that pushes you into things you aren't ready for. It lasted maybe a month and then he dumped me for my friend Suzie. I played cool and tough whenever I saw him, showing off my confidence like Julia Roberts in *Erin Brockovich*. But secretly, I wrote poems to try to heal my tragically broken heart.

All of my future relationships lasted less than three months. The defense mechanism in me is convinced that, not wanting to be dumped again, I'd only go for the safe friends as boyfriends and then break up with them after a short while because I didn't feel "that way" about them.

But that all changed with Chris.

Even though I knew he was trouble from the moment we met.

AN INTERESTING INTRODUCTION

Chris and I met in college the summer of 1991. We were both living in a dorm at The University of Texas. I don't remember what I was wearing, what the weather was like outside or what kind of mood I was in. I can't even recall why I walked into my friend's dorm room. But whatever the reason, it would inexorably change my life.

I opened the door to see a tall, handsome guy with a waist almost as small as mine and strong arms the size of my quads. He seemed perfectly at ease, leaning against a desk talking to Karmit and Liz, two freshmen who lived on my floor. Then the cute stranger with the bright blue eyes flashed me a boyish grin and asked, "Are you a virgin?"

What kind of pompous ass asks a question like that the first time he meets a girl? It's not like I was wearing a leather bustier and red stilettos. This is a dorm, not a strip club. But then, if it were a strip club, he wouldn't need to ask that question.

I left the room without another word, too speechless

to respond. What had they been talking about that led to that question? Should I be insulted or flattered? I'll admit he had me thinking about it—or him. I caught a glimpse of myself in the mirror to make sure I wasn't actually wearing a leather bustier.

FOR THE RECORD

Yes—the first question I asked my future wife when we met was, "Are you a virgin?" I'd like to think that I am different now. And I'd like to think that this start tells you how far I have come. But the truth is that from this start, it was her efforts that changed me; she made me tolerable.

The subject of sex had come up as it frequently does in the raging-hormone confines of a college dorm. We had been discussing whether or not it was possible for someone to be a virgin in college anymore. We wondered if it was even important.

The door to the dormitory swung open and a young, voluptuous, smooth skinned girl walked in. I was instantly attracted to her, like a moth to light. She had a mysterious energy that was emanating from her. It was seductive but somehow still innocent.

Part of me wanted to shock her, to grab her attention. I desperately wanted her to join the conversation, but I didn't know how to draw her in. So I blurted out the first words that came to mind. Naturally, it was the absolute wrong thing to ask.

Michelle didn't answer; she just stared at me and then blocked me out as if she was looking right through me. She was there to borrow an iron for a date. I thought she was going to take the iron to my face. Oh, did I have a lot of work to do.

LESSON 2: BE CAREFUL WHAT YOU SAY WHEN YOU FIRST MEET A GIRL. SHE COULD END UP BEING YOUR WIFE.

THE SOFTBALL GAME

The day after my first train wreck encounter with Chris, I was eating lunch in the cafeteria and noticed him at the end of our table, talking and laughing with his friends. There was something so irritating yet likeable about him. When Chris stood up to leave, he asked if anyone could give him a ride to the intramural fields.

Every floor of our dorm had a softball team and Floor 17, my team, had a game that afternoon. So when nobody else piped up, I offered to take him. I was curious. And if things went sour, I still had the iron in my back seat.

The entire car ride, he talked about going out with me, but I honestly couldn't tell if he was teasing or not so I wrote it off. Quite frankly, I felt he was out of my league. But later that night, he was waiting outside my dorm room upon my return from a date with Jeff—a guy who I might have considered my boyfriend by this time if someone had asked. Chris claimed to be very upset that I hadn't gone out with him. Would I make it up to him with a kiss? He pleaded with those big blue eyes. When I refused his request, he asked me for an innocent peck on the cheek. I leaned in and he surprised me by turning his head so our lips met. Cheeky bastard. He got the kiss he wanted.

As I warned, he was clearly trouble. But my heart was winning the intense battle with my mind. Every time I tried to resist him, my knees would buckle and I'd be swept up in his boyish charm. Ultimately, I fell for his supreme confidence and playful spirit.

A week after our first ride to the softball fields, it was time for our softball teams, both undefeated, to play against each other. Chris had been taunting me for several days, claiming that his team was going to kick my team's butt. He strutted around like a peacock, boasting about how superior his team was. I didn't believe a word he said.

I'd had a few hits (though if you ask Chris, he'd swear he got me out every time I was up), he'd had a few hits, and the score was tied in the eighth inning.

It was my turn to bat with the bases loaded and two outs. The heat was on. The wind up, pitch, and I swung with all my strength. The ball sailed through the air far past the outfielders. It was like *The Natural* without the exploding stadium lights. I sprinted around the bases and as I crossed home plate, my teammates lifted me on their shoulders, hooting and hollering.

In reality, it was one of the worst hits of my life. A nine-year-old schoolgirl could have hit the ball harder than I did. My slow dribbler went straight to the pitcher, who whipped around and launched it to first base—guarded by Chris—for the sure and final out. But the stars aligned somewhere out in the universe. Chris dropped the ball. Safe. Our team scored two runs and we pulled out the victory.

What Chris would admit later is that God was smiting him for being cocky. His fiendish plan was to catch the ball, saunter over a few steps in front of the base and have me plow straight into him for the out. He swears it was this rotten plan that made him drop the ball—that it never would have happened if he'd waited patiently on base like a sound baseball player should. Sounds like a whole lot of excuses if you ask me.

A SINGLE RED ROSE

After Michelle got over the shock of my initial question, we spent most of the summer together. I would come over to her dorm room and watch science class lessons with her. She would watch nearly every White Sox game with me.

I stole a kiss from her every once in a while, but other than these kisses and the constant sexual tension, our relationship was plutonic. I wasn't even sure that she felt the tension. Understanding a woman is like trying to make sense of the U.S. tax code—and I have an accounting degree.

Nonetheless, Michelle became my best friend. Simple and true.

She would join me on my late night snack excursions, even when it was two o'clock in the morning and the streets of West Campus were littered with drunken frat boys hoping to get some action. She'd spend time with me when I needed a friend. We'd go for long walks to talk about our goals and dreams. She was always honest with me. She was the first friend to ever tell me I probably needed to work harder to achieve all the dreams I had.

She told me when I was lazy, made sure I knew it when I was wrong and never let me slide when I was judging someone. But the best part is that I never minded when she told me these things. She wasn't trying to make me who she wanted me to be, just who I wanted to be. It was like I was talking to a part of me, the part of me that wanted to make me better at any cost.

Michelle was leaving for the second semester of the summer. She had plans for a vacation with her family and friends. The day she left for the airport, I got stuck waiting for my teacher's office hours after class. I rushed back to see if I could catch her before she left, but I was too late. It crushed me.

I climbed the stairs to my room, a thick wave of loneliness settled into my bones. I missed her already. My roommate was getting ready for a date, but he told me that Michelle had stopped by and left me something. I scurried over to my bed to find a present—a single red rose.

I had no idea what the colors of roses meant, but I knew how it made me feel. I wanted to be with her right then. A piece of me felt like it was missing. No one had ever given me something like that before. No one had ever meant this much to me before, and the worst part was for the next month, there was nothing I could do about it.

I fell back on my twin bed and twiddled the rose in my fingers, smelling the subtle scent, alone for now, but feeling more with someone than ever before. I missed her even more with every thought.

THE COLOSSAL MISCOMMUNICATION

I was very young when Chris and I started dating, and so with the first mention of marriage, I made it clear that we'd need to wait to talk about it until I turned 25. What Chris didn't understand was that on January 2nd, on my twenty-fifth birthday, I was ready for a ring on my finger.

He thought, "not talking about it," meant that we actually needed to start the dialogue then.

This was a colossal miscommunication.

What proceeded were a parade of gifts and vacations throughout the year that left me with no ring and a ballooning sense of panic. Each time I opened a new jewelry box it was like playing *Let's Make a Deal.* The vacations were worse—I had to play Nancy Drew and interpret his clues that always turned out to be red herrings.

Finally in October, it was time for a conversation that would reach in and yank my stomach contents up into my throat. But I needed an answer. So I asked the question, "Why don't you want to marry me?" Then I heard the dreaded words that made my heart shatter into a million pieces as if it had been frozen in dry ice and then thrown to the unforgiving pavement ten stories below.

"I'm not ready. I need more time."

More time! How can he need more time? We'd known each other for seven years!

Chris asked how long he had before I'd leave him. I begrudgingly gave him one more year.

THE SURPRISE

When we were graduating college, Michelle told me that she wanted to wait until she was 25 to talk about marriage. I had asked her, in passing, to marry me several times by then. I was pretty sure in college that she was the one, but I want people to get what they want, especially her. So I waited.

The problem is that the day she turned 25, she literally expected a ring. She might try to tell you she said she wanted to WAIT until she was 25, but what she said was that she did not want to DISCUSS getting married until she turned 25.

So on her birthday, she was clearly expecting to hold out a ring and I was expecting to have a conversation about it. I asked, "Don't we need to discuss it?" staying true to the agreement we had. The discussion was incredibly brief and unbeknownst to me our agreement was hurled out the window. Michelle said she was ready to be engaged.

But that just wouldn't do. I wanted our engagement to be special. I wanted it to be a fairytale. This was the woman of my dreams, the future mother of my children, my best friend and someone I chose to spend the rest of my life with. Forcing the engagement now would have been like passing up the Four Seasons in favor of Motel 6.

This moment, this event, had to be unique. I couldn't just ask her to marry me. I had to make her feel the way she had made me feel for the past seven years. So I set in motion an intricately constructed plan over the course of the next year to make it unforgettable.

I should take a moment here to make a confession. I am normally very disorganized, I procrastinate, there are countless projects that I begin but leave incomplete and I am not always thorough. But I had a fierce determination that our engagement would not be that way. My ingenious plan went like this: I would take her on several surprise trips throughout the year to throw her off. And then in December, when she was least expecting it, I would drop the big one on her. It was all smoke and mirrors up until then. I knew I was going to be walking a fine line so I told her sister the entire plan. Laura was my safety net in case my plan backfired. I just had to hope that she thought I was good enough for her little sister or else my surprise would go up in smoke.

The plan went like clockwork. First stop: Spain. I brought two of my friends to make sure that she did not think this would be THE trip. Surprise is one thing. Teasing is another. Michelle seemed very patient.

At the same time I started working on the ring. This had to be the crown jewel. Michelle had fallen in love with the jewelry designer, Cathy Waterman, and I set out to ask Cathy to make a setting for a perfect stone.

Picking the stone had become an adventure in and of itself. I learned enough about diamonds to become a gemologist. I read books and online articles, went to diamond stores and consulted friends. I finally found "the one"—the princess diamond that would be my companion when I got on one knee. I nicknamed the ring Cathy. If Michelle said no, at least I had Cathy to lean on.

Throughout the summer and into the fall, I continued working on the ring. But I sensed that I was running out of time. Michelle was quietly growing impatient. In October, we planned a long weekend to San Francisco. To ease her frustration, I surprised Michelle with Cathy Waterman—earrings, that is. When she opened the box, I watched her smile deflate like a balloon. The earrings had pushed her over the edge.

When we returned home, she asked me point blank if I was really ever going to marry her. I felt horrible.

I had the stone in a drawer just five feet away. I could have whipped open the box and ended this whole mess in an instant. But I didn't want to ruin the surprise. I assured her that I just needed a little more time. Crisis avoided. I felt horrible, like I was torturing her, but I wanted to finish it, so I went in the other room to get an update on my project with Ms. Waterman.

By December, all of the pieces were finally in place. I'd asked Michelle's father for his permission to marry his daughter during our trip to Miami over Thanksgiving, to which he'd replied, "We would be excited to have you as part of the family."

Blessing—check.

Ring—almost check. It was supposed to arrive in a few days.

The big show was ready to go on.

I had dropped subtle hints to Michelle on several occasions that I really wanted to get away one more time before the end of the year. We had been working at a feverish pace at a startup and it wasn't unusual for me to want to go on a trip out of the blue to blow off steam. So a few days before the trip, I told her that I'd booked us two tickets for a vacation—the destination a secret.

The morning of the flight, with the ring securely in my jacket pocket, Michelle and I headed to the airport, my plans and my secret intact. I'd never worked on any project this long in my life. I felt like a conman pulling off the heist of a lifetime.

Michelle's sister called that morning—Laura was

planning to meet us in the airport in Dallas on our way through. Since she was working at American Airlines at the time, that was logical enough. But when her mom called too, I begged her not to answer it. The more things out of the norm, the more I risked blowing my surprise.

The flight to Paris felt excruciatingly long. Michelle will tell you that I slept and she barely got a wink in, but that is revisionist history. I was drowning in nerves, too anxious to sleep. Instead, I watched Michelle while she slept, her chest gently rising and falling. At one point the flight attendant said she looked like a princess. My heart fluttered with joy.

We arrived first thing in the morning and headed to the Ritz. I had planned on asking her the next day but I knew I couldn't wait. In my mind I came up with a million reasons to do it today, same date as my brother's birthday, Friday would be less crowded at Versailles, we had a dinner reservation the next evening that was early. But the truth is my nerves were frayed and I wanted it done. Excitement was pulsing through my veins. So I asked her to take a shower and get ready.

She didn't want to go. She was tired. And it was cold and raining outside.

I gave her no choice.

She grumbled.

On the train ride out to Versailles, Michelle dozed, while I felt the ring burn a whole in my pocket. At least twice I checked to make sure it was still there. Michelle woke just as the train rolled into the station. We moseyed along the street to the castle in the misty rain.

When we arrived, I asked Michelle to take a few steps out into the gardens so I could get her picture. I really wanted a picture before and after the moment. But she defiantly refused (something about it being cold, her hat looking funny and that I was being like her mother who always wants to take pictures, blah, blah, blah).

If you ask her now she will admit that she was being a bitch.

If you ask me now, I will agree.

After incessantly begging, cajoling and pleading, she finally caved. The pictures were priceless, especially the one with her tongue sticking out.

The moment was here. Pictures taken, I got on one knee and completed my quest.

I could tell by Michelle's face that she had no idea. When I began to kneel she looked first confused and then she lit up like a firecracker, completely surprised. The extra work, the whole project, was worth it. The icy rain seemed to melt around us.

Somewhere in all the jubilant tears, hugs and kisses, she finally whispered a single, beautiful word. Yes.

LESSON 3: SPECIAL MEMORIES LAST A LIFETIME.

PARIS—THE CITY OF LOVE

In December, Chris said he needed a getaway from work. He wanted it to be a surprise, so he would not disclose the destination. I was given only the approximate temperature for packing purposes. I wonder if this is how wild animals feel when they are captured.

Had he not thoroughly convinced me that he wasn't ready to marry me (with those heart-shattering words), I would not have let down my Nancy Drew guard. But it never even crossed my mind that this was the surprise engagement trip I'd been secretly hoping for since the beginning of the year. No more *Let's Make a Deal* jewelry boxes. This was the big one.

When he got down on one knee in the enchanting gardens of Versailles, I was stunned. And apparently speechless, since Chris claims it took me an eternity to say yes. My floodgate of tears, hugs, and kisses didn't answer the question? He gently slid the ring on my finger and a big grin bloomed on my face. I was over the moon.

I never would have thought four words could make me so happy. The stinging cold rain no longer bothered me. We frolicked through the gardens, taking pictures and then warmed up with the best cup of hot chocolate we'd ever tasted. Most girls dream of having a fairytale love story. This was mine.

I DO

Our engagement was not followed by a quick wedding. I have several valid reasons, though now that I had a sparkling diamond on my finger, I wasn't in a huge rush to get hitched. I'm sure all of those movies about gaggles of girls dreaming of their wedding day are accurate for some, but that just isn't me. Actually, I never envisioned my wedding day. Not even in a dream.

My sister got engaged just a few months after I did and figuring my parents would not want us planning two weddings at once, Chris and I sat back and waited our turn. Then the same happened with Chris' older sister. Meanwhile, the high tech market was keeping us both very busy with work.

When the tech bubble burst, everything finally fell perfectly into place. In April 2002, after dating since the first Bush was president and being engaged since the Clinton Administration, Chris and I were married.

I'd asked that our engagement be special, and Chris

delivered on his promise. Our wedding weekend carried on the tradition of storybook perfection.

At our Rehearsal Dinner, Laura conjured up a bellowing laughter from the audience by telling a story about Chris. In a nutshell, she was able to name at least twenty professions—starting with major league baseball player and ending with a spy—that Chris had mentioned wanting to pursue in the ten years she had known him. Always an impulsive dreamer. (The list hasn't grown much since then. Being a marine is a new one, mostly because of Chris' younger brother Jake who is in Iraq as I type these words.)

Speaking of Jake, he one-upped my sister by announcing at the end of his speech that, "Unlike my brother, I am, in fact, a spy." He had the audience rolling.

When it was my turn, I got so choked up talking about Chris I had to skip over him altogether. Everyone but Chris thought that was endearing.

Chris, who swears he can control the weather, scared away the rain that had been grumbling all week. That was a really good thing, because our venue was outdoors at the French Legation, a tiny white house surrounded by a few acres of landscaped grounds and a timeless stone wall. In the background is a sprawling panoramic view of the capital building and downtown Austin. The ambiance would have been ruined under big white tents and sheets of rain.

On our wedding day, the weather was perfect—sunny and not too warm. The butterflies fluttered in the air all around us. The orchestra played beautifully while I walk down the rose-petaled aisle. I didn't trip. We exchanged our vows and rings and I exhaled for the first time as a married woman. The dinner and wedding cakes were scrumptious. Everyone danced, imbibed with his or her drink of choice. Jake enjoyed four bottles of champagne and performed on stage with the band. He would make a good spy.

Our wedding was such a magical experience that I didn't want it to end. I was swept up in all the romance. When it was time for our exit, we were greeted by a cloud of bubbles and a procession of friends and family. It all went too fast and I was sad to say goodbye.

EXPECTATIONS

Here we are almost three years later, ready for a new chapter in our lives. We are trying for a baby. I am looking forward to the moment when I hold a positive pregnancy test in my hand and know that I am going to be a mom. Chris is excited about the unlimited sex. But he is convinced that I will get pregnant the very first month as a cruel joke to rain on his sex parade. I figure it will take about eight months—the same amount of time it took my sister and mother to get pregnant with their first. So we place a bet to see who's closest.

Statistics say there's a 20% chance in any one month that a healthy couple will achieve a pregnancy and carry it to term. Of course, those chances vary with age. If I were in my twenties, the average would be five monthly cycles, but women in their early thirties will get pregnant, on average, after nine cycles. So I'm being pretty realistic in hoping I'm just about average.

THE MILLER CURSE

You've heard stories of curses. Our family has its own, which my brother and I have termed "The Miller Curse." Our curse is that our family's lives are rarely straightforward. Things we think are a shoe-in never happen the way you expect them to.

You know how in great movies, everything usually works itself out but in an unexpected way? That's typical for us.

In college I really wanted to graduate from the UT business school. Jobs were hard to come by, but the accounting program was the best in the country and therefore if you had an accounting degree you got a job.

I started college off, let's just say slowly, and needed to make really good grades to be able to take classes in the business school. But after trying as hard as I could, I ended up one hundredth of a point below the required GPA. So my circuitous route began. I spent months talking to the professors, administrators and deans, until one Christmas Eve I received a letter from Dean Witt, granting me an exception and confirming my entrance into the business school. I had become the exception.

Much of my life has been spent being the exception.

It's a spring day and Michelle and I have agreed to start trying. She's beaming like the sun, as am I. I put the worries of the long-term responsibility of a child out of my mind. First things first—we have to try, we have to get pregnant and then we have to have the baby. Responsibility comes later, right?

I'm also overjoyed about the 'trying' process. Trying is code for oodles of sex. But with my luck, she'll get pregnant within a month. The trying phase will be over and my sexcapades will come to an end. I guess she'd notice if I slipped on a condom.

Michelle and I make a wager on how long it will take before she is pregnant. The over/under is six months. I take the under. I figure betting on my bad luck is a smart move. And either way, I should be happy, right?

LESSON 4: SOMETIMES EVEN I DON'T UNDERSTAND HOW THE MILLER CURSE WILL PLAY OUT.

TIME TO START A FAMILY

I arrive at my annual visit to the OB/GYN and for the first time since I was old enough to start getting Pap smears, I'm actually happy to be there. In the waiting area, I pretend to peruse through some *Highlights* magazines while secretly spying a mother playing with her baby.

I patiently wait for the doctor in a cold examination room, barely covered by a thin purple gown. I look down and realize I'm (barely) covered in clowns. Who designs these and why do they insist on making you feel five years old?

Dr. Gunter arrives with a big grin, shakes my hand and before she can even ask a question, I spill the news that we want to start trying for a baby. She's the first person I've told because Chris talked me into keeping it a secret from our families for now.

"Well, congratulations!" she says.

It feels even more official now that someone else knows. I feel a flutter in my stomach. I'm tempted to barrel out after the appointment and raid the nearby Babies-R-Us for some soft baby blankets, a set of onesies in blue and pink, and those teeny, tiny socks that turn on the waterworks every time I see them.

My elation is crushed seconds later, however, when I find out Dr. Gunter is no longer delivering babies. (Something about twenty years being far too long to deal with calls in the middle of the night.) I've been seeing her since my first year in college fifteen years ago. I've known her longer than I've known Chris. I trust her.

I'd seen a too-close-for-comfort look at my sister's first delivery—a 16-hour ordeal. It was a circus show. When I think about the craziness of the labor process, I had always pictured Dr. Gunter's gentle face, warm voice and calm manor helping me through it all. Chris isn't the pep talking coach I was looking for, but he'll be right by my side cracking jokes and doing everything he can to make me laugh. I'm not sure how he can make me laugh through the ordeal of labor, but I'll be interested to see him try.

"Is there anything I need to know now that we're trying?" I ask before I leave (besides, 'who the heck is going to deliver my baby? Thanks for leaving me doc.'). She hands me a laundry list of foods to stay away from that could be harmful to a fetus and a preconception checklist. I also receive a white baggy full of prenatal vitamins to try. I feel like a kid at Halloween. But instead of the end result being a cavity, I'm getting a bun in my oven.

So that's it. I have my plan. Throw the birth control pills away. Have sex. Take prenatal vitamins. Stay away from certain foods. Don't change the cat litter. Get pregnant. No problem.

Chris requests elaborate seductions every night. Kinky outfits. Body butter and oils (what am I, a piece of toast?). Extra special treats. He's milking this opportunity for all it's worth. Especially since he truly believes that the powers upstairs will only allow him one month of joy.

Also, I think our cats, Tigger and Puck, are onto us. They are trying to thwart our baby-making plans by sprawling on the bed and meowing loudly. When the crying doesn't get our attention, they leap to the top of our stainless steel canopy and perform a high wire walk around the frame. Tigger goes one way, Puck goes the other, and they meet in the middle and look down at us.

When I promptly lock them out so that Chris and I can get down to business, they try a different tactic. We live in a small 1,400 square foot house that's arranged in roughly a circle and you can walk either way to get to any one of the rooms. Not a minute later, they are at the door, clawing and scratching. When I open one door and shoo them away, they both run to the other door and begin again.

We learn to ignore them.

It's day ten of my cycle and we have our first challengers seeking an egg. Chris encourages them to swim, swim, swim. I add, "But conserve some of that energy, because you guys only have five days to live—if you're lucky!"

It's a strange experience actually; when sex means something more than passion or pleasure or love. I didn't think I would feel any different, but I do. There's a bit more pressure than your every-day-fooling-around. On the flip side, it also feels more meaningful to me. It's the beginning of possibility.

Days eleven through fifteen continue the antics— Chris taking advantage of my need of him and the cats trying to sabotage our plans, meowing on the dresser, peeking under the doors and just being generally annoying.

Now all we can do is wait. And take vitamins. And maybe do a little rain dance. And hope that one of Chris' boys will find the golden egg.

Chris and I had agreed to not keep track of the days and just roll with it for a while. We are at dinner when our friends announce they are pregnant. Chris asks our friend David, "Isn't it awesome? All the sex you want?"

David proceeds to shatter Chris' dreams with his answer. "Well, it was at first, but then Jennifer read up on it and put all these rules in place. It went from fun every day to two days a month."

All Jennifer can do is shrug in agreement. But hey, they're pregnant, so they must have done something right.

Chris is adorable, talking to my stomach every day just in case there's a baby boy or girl growing inside of me. My trial of several prenatal vitamins has twisted my stomach into a rope swing, so I'm not sure if the nausea is from the pills or pregnancy hormones.

When the cramps do come, I'm only slightly disappointed. I never expected it would happen the first month.

We have lift-off. We just don't have a baby to accompany us on our ship yet.

TWO MONTHS IN

Michelle and I are lying in bed late one Saturday morning, the sun streaming through the blinds, dappling the room in warm light. We're enjoying being flat-out lazy and hanging out with our dozy cats.

Michelle mentions that it's been two months of trying and still nothing. I've been taking full advantage of the process, being seduced even when I haven't wanted to be seduced (I never thought that was possible before this). I've made her work for it because I figured it wouldn't last long. It's not like I've been holding back. I have been trying. But now I am feeling guilty because trying so far hasn't worked for shit.

I turn and face her. I tell her sincerely that it will happen; it just might take some time. She smiles but doesn't reply. I'm certain that she is not replying because she never wants to get her hopes up. Her eyes, those big brownies glowing in the sun, tell me she doesn't want to set herself up for disappointment.

I'm okay with this. But I still want to give her hope. So I earnestly repeat that it will all work out. I am sure of it. And if it doesn't, then we will travel all over the world and borrow other people's kids for the fun stuff. We'll just trade them in for a new one when they break (or whine), like our humidifier from Target. She smiles, but not big enough. Not with her eyes.

Will it happen next month, or the month after that? Or is there something we don't know?

LESSON 5: THE WAITING SEEMS LIKE THE HARDEST PART.

FREEBIES AND FRUSTRATION

At the end of January, Chris agreed I could tell people we were trying. It felt like progress sharing the news with family and friends—as if telling people what we were hoping for might just make it come true.

We are only a few months into the process and we weren't supposed to start trying until this month anyway, so the last two months I consider freebies. Everything still feels shiny and new. And I am a woman on a mission. Being "in the mood" is no longer an ingredient in the master recipe. Neither headaches nor stomach aches nor exhaustion can stop me. I'm an Easy-Bake oven ready to bake the goods. If it's anywhere close to the right time, I'll acquiesce (or more often, be the designated seductress). It's funny how our roles have swapped. While Chris was almost always the lone wolf hungry for sex, now it is my turn to pounce.

To give you a rough idea of the lengths Chris will go to for sex, he once presented me with an article from *Maxim Magazine* on the sexual activities of couples, as if this piece of "literature" was the bible on all things sex. He pranced around, proud of his brilliant research find. It proceeded to suggest absurd statistics, such as the average couple has sex twice a day (yeah if you are an Olympic gymnast), oral sex is doled out as often as trinkets at a tech conference and that swallowing provides negative calories just like grapefruit juice. But Chris, per usual, glossed over the details and missed a crucial point. He'd neglected to see the fine print at the top where it suggested that men provide this (highly) fictional list to their significant others to convince them they needed to ratchet it up in the sex department. I wasn't buying it. I'm a woman—I know how to spot a fake.

Four days down and only one more to go for this cycle. One thing I've learned already is that with the pressure of trying, waiting until midnight to fool around isn't always the best strategy. So today, I'll try to pounce early.

Chris slumps in the door and by the look on his face, I can tell I'm in for a challenge. He's had a frustrating day at work and can't stop talking about it. This isn't a typical bad day—this is a colossally terrible day.

Luckily, all it takes is one change of an outfit to alter Chris' mood. Maybe that patience and extra effort will make a difference. Can't a girl dream? Now it is ten days of waiting again until we find out if this is the magical month.

Nine days later, my dream is crushed again.

OFFICIALLY TRYING

We're officially allowed to tell people we're trying. Now this isn't really a big deal to me; my list is very short. I mainly want to tell my family and a few close friends.

My brother Jake, who is in the Marines and in Iraq responds, "You go boy!" Ten years ago he would have asked, "So I guess you get to have sex?" Very little has changed.

My younger sister Heather, who I think of as the

brilliant, quiet one, tells me we will make excellent parents. Funny. I feel that I might just screw this up worse than anything ever.

My older sister is very excited, and her husband tells her to tell me, "Congrats on the sex, you're on your own for the other part." Lorie just tells me she is happy for me.

My mother, a high school soccer coach, is probably the most excited about our news. This would be her first grandkid and she's ready. She loves her "soccer girls" and one of my favorite mental images of her is teaching my kids to play the game that she loves.

I would describe my father as a gentle giant, but one who you don't want to piss off. When he's mad, he reminds me of Clint Eastwood—he doesn't need words to get his point across. I tell him on the phone and he responds the quickest and loudest. "Hey, that's great." He has this ability to be truly, genuinely happy for others. Years of putting his four kids' happiness first must have drilled this into him.

I also tell my best friends Dan and Dustin over beers one night. All I remember is that I didn't pay for drinks and I threw up in the cab on the way home. Dan was the designated non-drunk and he ended up negotiating our exit fee with the cab driver. Thanks Dan.

I was in no shape to try for kids that night.

LESSON 6: CELEBRATING "TRYING TO GET PREGNANT" WITH LOTS OF ALCOHOL MAY NOT EXACTLY HELP WITH YOUR GOAL.

SCHEDULES AND PEE STICKS

I am now saying the one thing that I thought I would never say. But sex isn't much fun anymore. *What the hell am I talking about? What's happened to me?*

You are never going to see my wife naked, but she looks incredible, especially naked. In fact, it used to be that just the thought of her naked was enough for me. That was until this whole regiment began.

It could be the pressure, or the cats always hanging around waiting for the show, but somehow it's not fun anymore. It just seems like we're doing it for someone else.

On a typical workday, I walk in the door and Michelle is ready to go for a walk. We head out into the neighborhood, where we do an hour loop, talking about everything until my mind wanders off and the pressures of the day fade away with the sun. Then we work our way through showers, eating dinner and, when we feel like it, having sex, not necessarily in that order.

Today when I came home from work, Michelle was nowhere in sight. I drop off my backpack and go searching for her, pausing briefly to pet our two cats. Puck trails behind me, nipping at my heels. In our bedroom,

I lose the work clothes and slip on my workout clothes.

I head to the bathroom calling her name, and find her peeing on a stick. This isn't the sexiest thing I have ever witnessed. It's the equivalent of hearing a girl fart. And it's an image I don't need implanted in my mind with all the other thoughts rummaging around in my brain.

I've heard about the <u>ovulation tests</u> before, but this is the first time I've seen it. Suddenly a stick determines our agenda for the night. I get from the goofy commercial that "this is the most advanced piece of technology you will ever pee on," but it shouldn't act like my parole officer.

The stick tells Michelle she is <u>ovulating</u>. I am in luck. Only suddenly, I am not in the mood. What has happened to me? I am ALWAYS in the mood.

Things have changed. Sex is now about pee sticks and research. Suddenly a "schedule" becomes very important. Did I mention that I vehemently detest schedules and planning and deadlines? It stresses me out. And now I've figured out it kills my sex drive like a cheetah taking down a hobbled gazelle.

"Ready for a walk?" I ask. Michelle looks at me with her seductive brown eyes. Being not in the mood makes this pretty uncomfortable. Did I mention that my defense mechanism for uncomfortable feelings is comedy? I laugh.

Those doughy brown eyes turn to scorn. Clearly, laughing wasn't the response she was looking for. I open my mouth to explain, and then leave it gaping, not knowing what to say.

So I flash her a smile. Michelle wills her eyes seductive again. My smile is perhaps a bit too big. She glares at me, puzzled. I glance down at Puck, he chirps and then pads out of the room. He can tell this isn't going well.

I ask her, "Can we walk first?"

Her face flickers a sign of disappointment. I've blown it. Puck was right.

"Okay," Michelle replies.

About three miles in, when I hope she is too tired to make fun of me, I admit that I wasn't in the mood. A wide smile cracks across her face.

"Oh really? This from someone who swears he is ALWAYS in the mood!"

Her smile lights up my world. She is so beautiful when she smiles. If only it weren't at my expense.

"Yes," and then I quickly add, "but you can't make fun of me because I told you. Don't punish me for honesty."

At this, she giggles. It's deliciously sexy. Then she says, "I guess I'll just have to help you out then."

And just like that, I'm in the mood again.

LESSON 7: I'M EASY.

READY AND WAITING

Michelle and I are on a walk through our neighborhood. We walk through a park and there happen to be several kids playing on the playground. A brother and a sister are "helping" each other with gentle shoves. One tries to shove gum in the other's hair. They swing on the monkey bars, pounce at each other on the playscape and scurry through the gravel in chase. Another child is learning to bounce a ball underneath the basketball hoop. He bends to pick it up, but kicks it accidentally. It rolls toward us.

I bound over and pick it up. He stops, looking up with a shy smile; I smile and roll it back. He goes back to bouncing, forgetting he ever lost it.

Remember how I wasn't sure I was ready for kids yet? There are a lot of kids in the world and all of them are doing cool stuff. Not just at the playground. I recently saw a mother and daughter at the airport and I listened as she taught her daughter how to say the word kitty, one syllable at a time.

They say that absence makes the heart grow fonder. This is true, but I think that it's also true that time brings out what is truly in your heart. And my heart now tells me that I really want to have a child. I look forward to teaching my daughter or son everything I know, and all the things I don't know that we can learn together.

I should have agreed to start sooner. I should never have waited. We still don't have any money and what the hell is the difference? What did I accomplish by waiting? Nothing.

I'm worried that my hesitation has caused the problem. I'm incredibly superstitious. I got it from my baseball playing days. Or you could say I believe firmly in my own version of Schrödinger's cat. The theory goes like this: if you had a cat in a box and you broke a vial that contained either poison or harmless liquid, then until you opened the box, the cat is both alive and dead. In my twisted brain, I've distorted this to mean that knowing or not knowing, wanting or not wanting, somehow affects the outcome.

And in this case, I think I could have jinxed us because I wasn't ready.

LESSON 8: SUPERSTITIONS AROUND CONCEIVING SOUND JUST AS INSANE AS WEARING THE SAME BOXERS TO EVERY SPORTING EVENT.

FERTILITY STEPS

Once everyone knew we had been trying for a while without succeeding, we were on the receiving end of a lot of unsolicited advice. First and foremost was to make sure I knew when I was ovulating—i.e. when my body would release an egg from my ovary. AKA the "pee stick" test. Actually, there are two versions of peeing on a stick: ovulation predictor kits and home pregnancy tests.

Over-the-counter <u>ovulation predictor kits</u> help pinpoint your most fertile time of the month—the day before ovulation and the day of ovulation. (Remember what we said in the prologue—if you want more information about any word, head to the back of this book for definitions in Appendix A.) How does it work? It measures the <u>Luteinizing hormone</u>, or LH in your urine, which increases dramatically 24-48 hours before ovulation. This hormone is actually what triggers the ovulation process to begin. So, having sex during the 24 hours following this surge maximizes your chances of getting pregnant. Most importantly, those kits tell you IF you are ovulating—a key component to getting pregnant. No ovulation = no eggs = no embryos = no baby!

The most common female infertility factor is an <u>ovulation disorder</u>. If you aren't ovulating, there are myriad ways to solve that problem, from fertility medications to moving your bed under a window where the moonlight can seep through (I couldn't make this stuff up if I tried, although the latter sounds more for werewolves if you ask me). But if the test shows a surge each month, then you can at least put a check mark next to that item.

The ovulation sticks came into play after four months of trying on our own. Our friend David was right—once you go down the path of fertility research, you can kiss the fun and spontaneity goodbye. And the pressure begins to mount too. Even Chris wasn't so excited about the extra action anymore. That is saying a lot.

FERTILITY FISH AND OTHER ADVICE

We're seven months in. No matter what crazy lengths we go to, at the end of every cycle the cramps came and hope dissolves into disappointment. I'm a bad news first person. The bad news is that 80% of couples trying to conceive are pregnant by now. This is definitely one of those times I'd prefer not to be in the minority. The good news is, research shows that 50% of couples that have tried to conceive for six months without success will conceive in the next six months without any special treatment. I keep telling myself that it will happen eventually.

The list of advice continues with the passing months. Avoiding strenuous exercise (I gave up Bodhi Yoga and soccer). No caffeine (luckily I'd already given that up long ago). Trying acupuncture and their bitter herbs and teas. Tracking my basal body temperature (pretty much the same goal as the ovulation predictor kits in determining when you are ovulating, though acupuncturists also like to check out the charts to see if your temperatures are warm enough after ovulation to sustain a pregnancy). Positioning during, positioning after, how much time to wait before getting out of bed (you don't want all of the sperm going the wrong way), etc. It's not proven that a handstand will help the sperm travel to their destination, but it doesn't hurt to try (unless you fall down). Welcome to the circus.

"Oh, you might want to try taking Robitussin for five days before you ovulate," my sister suggests. I'm not sniffling. What does cough syrup have to do with fertility? I Google it and discover that Robitussin helps to loosen and thin cervical mucous just like it would loosen the phlegm in your chest, which means the sperm have a smooth fluid in which to swim toward their target. Sorry sperm, I didn't realize my vaginal canal could be as muddy as The Mississippi, making it hard to swim. I take Robitussin to see if it makes a difference.

My sister also came to Austin bearing fertility gifts.

First was a bottle of fertility pills, which her housekeeper swore by after trying to conceive on her own for two years and then getting pregnant within a couple of months of taking them. I look at it skeptically, but then start popping them like M&M'S. My stomach is a mess the next day and I spend nearly all afternoon on the toilet, trying to cleanse my body of those wretched pills. Thanks sis.

The second gift was the most absurd looking statue that is perched on my nightstand right now, watching over us while we sleep. Its glowing eyes stare at me in a scary, totally non-comforting way. It's called a <u>Fertility Fish</u>. It looks like a trinket you'd buy half-drunk at a gift shop in Cancun during spring break. Actually, it was a gift from her mother-in-law when they were ready to have kids. Now this thing has become something of a family heirloom.

When Laura had mentioned the Fertility Fish in the past, I pictured a little glass or ceramic fish that fits in the palm of your hand or something you'd place under your pillow. This foreign object isn't remotely close to what I'd imagined. It's a red stained wooden, African-looking relic, about twelve inches high and three inches wide with a clattering bell around the neck. I don't know much about it except that it's supposed to bring fertility luck. Check out the picture below so you can pick one up for yourself the next time you're drunk south of the border.

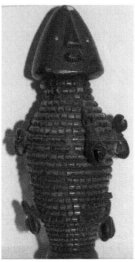

The Fertility Fish

It was even suggested, quite often actually, that we try getting drunk. A few friends we spoke with said after months and months of trying, they got pregnant after she got totally sloshed at exactly the right time of the month for fooling around.

The thing is, I don't feel any pressure or stress at this point. I'm not super frustrated. I'm not pulling my hair out. I don't have any negative thoughts (okay, maybe a tiny pin prick in my brain thinks 'What if we don't ever get pregnant?'). I just figure these things take time, and drunken debauchery isn't going to solve anything. One day, when our baby is crying in the middle of the night and I've had an hour of sleep, at least I'll think, 'So this is what we tried so hard for!' with a big grin, instead of 'Why oh why did I want to have children?'

I let most of the advice we receive roll off my shoulders and keep on, keeping on...

IT'S MY FAULT

I am being as supportive as I can be, but I'm feeling guilty about the excesses I'm getting when Michelle coerces me. We're about to begin the next round of trying.

I'm distracted, perhaps by Puck who is crying at the door. I decide in my wisdom to just open the door. What's the worst he can do?

It could also be that there is a red sculpture on the nightstand next to the bed. It's a large red carved sculpture with bells on it, the Fertility Fish. I try to put it out of my mind, kissing Michelle, working on my part.

Suddenly my butt really tickles, so I scratch it, tell myself it is my imagination. It's my mind trying to distract me so I ignore it and go back to my job. A few seconds later I feel something tickling my butt again, but this time I am sure it is not my imagination.

Michelle asks me, "What?" I can tell she is worried I'm suddenly not in the mood.

"Something is tickling me."

I turn to look, and Puck is lying on the bed purring with his tail twitching expectantly back and forth across my butt. Michelle peeks around me and begins to laugh.

Damn cat. Serves me right for opening the door. I lunge toward him; he leaps across the bed and perches on the nightstand. I lunge for him again and he scurries off the nightstand and my motion bumps the nightstand, knocking the fertility fish to the floor. At this point Michelle and I are both laughing hysterically.

"Whatever happens this month, it's definitely my fault. I apologize in advance. The fertility fish and the cats clearly will not be rooting for us."

What can I do?

The good news is that hearing my wife laugh has put me firmly in the mood. At least something is easy.

LESSON 9: LET THE LITTLE THINGS MAKE YOU LAUGH.

ACUPUNCTURE

It's the middle of the night and I can't sleep. I tip toe upstairs and get online. Several people have mentioned trying <u>acupuncture</u> to help with fertility. I've been meaning to do some research and now seems as good a time as any. An hour later, I've decided it's certainly worth trying.

My acupuncturist, recommended by our friend Dan, is exactly what I pictured before walking in—a smart, kind, tiny Chinese man in his 50s. While I know he's speaking English, it sounds an awful lot like Chinese, so I haven't a clue what he is saying most of the time. Mostly, I smile and nod my head.

On my first visit, he asks me a lot of questions about my fertility status—what we've tried, what we know, etc. It's a pretty short conversation since we don't know much.

Having never tried acupuncture before, it takes some getting used to. Some needles I don't feel, but others make me wince when he taps them in. And since I don't follow his broken English, I'm not always ready for the pricks from head to toe. I'm supposed to relax my mind, so I close my eyes and try to drift off to sleep.

Usually it doesn't work. All I can think about is the long needles protruding out of my skin. But some days I'm so tired, I'm out before he's even closed the door.

I schedule appointments weekly and keep my fingers crossed that the needles are working their magic and will help me get pregnant.

GOD HAS A PLAN

Most people can't help but give you advice.

"Try relaxing." That one is the most common (and painfully obvious). Awesome—thanks. I could be a Buddhist monk and it wouldn't change a thing. Or would it? A friend of ours with fertility issues moved from the big city to the country and two months later—bam!— she was pregnant. The only change she made was slowing her lifestyle down. Maybe they're right.

There is the "get drunk" idea. There are two minor problems with this (besides not wanting to tell my future kid that he/she is the product of a drunken stupor). First, Michelle doesn't drink. Second, drinking is bad for the fertility process. For women, drinking can hinder the ovulation process. For men, drinking lowers the sperm count. And it doesn't naturally select for the weaker ones. It just kills at random.

There could be some truth to this approach on the female side. It's possible that it relaxes the woman, loosens her mucous, and just makes things a little bit easier. All possible, but not likely to make the required difference.

You've already heard about the fertility fish, which is either next to our bed or sometimes on the floor. It's been there for months now and nothing has changed. To its credit, it has the same success rate as the doctors do and it costs far less. My money is on the fish. It's also a nice reminder that there are lots of people rooting for us.

Lots of people tell us, "It will happen." They say it so matter-of-fact, as if all of our efforts are futile and we should just wait for a visit from an angel ala Joseph and Mary. Michelle doesn't appreciate these comments as much as I do. To be fair, they care enough to try and encourage, but they aren't insulting enough to think that they know more about the process than we do. They respect us and offer the one token thing they can: hope.

"Whatever happens is meant to be," or "God has a plan." I can accept the former. But I don't think that God's plan has anything to do with my testes or Michelle's uterus. And by the way, I don't mind if God does have this in his plan. I won't blame him either way.

Some of our closest friends have just stated plainly that we have to be able to have kids because we would make great parents. I want to believe we would make great parents and I will leave it at that. And I appreciate the compliment. There isn't anything I can think of that would be more important than being a good parent.

LESSON 10: KEEP THE FAITH. IN WHATEVER YOU BELIEVE IN. IT'S YOURS AND NO ONE CAN TAKE IT AWAY.

NEW RULES

Michelle has been peeing on loads of sticks. I could build a bonfire with all the sticks she has tinkled on (though the plastic would probably not be good tinder). Again, the result determines if we have sex or not. It's funny because this process truly is trying, in the other meaning of the word.

I am traveling tomorrow and according to her pee stick, tomorrow should be one of our windows. I've been traveling a lot and Michelle is starting to get concerned. It's tough to have sex when I'm out of town. I offer to have phone sex with her. Silence on the other end.

Based on Michelle's fertility research, one of the new "rules" is that I need to save my sperm for the two days before ovulation in order to have the best sperm count when the time comes. My boys have to be good and strong for The Mighty Mississippi.

Only one sperm has to make its weary way to one egg. Sperm, however, do not live forever. In fact, they typically live for only a few days. And there is only a 24-hour window in which the egg is ready to receive the sperm. Hence the reason that you want to conserve your sperm for the right time, when the egg has just released.

Now when everything is working perfectly, you don't have to worry about sperm counts and all this timing stuff. But since you're reading this book, everything may not be working perfectly.

So your sex life is now regimented for at least part of the month, by a plastic stick or a temperature change.

On top of this is the fact that when it is time, the man is required to perform. Which causes more stress. It's a call to arms that is sometimes hard to deliver on.

LESSON 11: TAKE WHAT YOU CAN GET. AND BE HAPPY ABOUT IT.

I CAN'T WAIT TO MEET YOU

Summer is winding down and Chris is traveling for work. It's month eight and I'm on cycle day 28 without any sign of cramps, which would be normal for most women, but is four days late for me. And I've felt a little nauseous over the last few days. So the plan is to take a pregnancy test tomorrow when Chris gets back in town. Could this finally be the month? My heart pounds just thinking about the possibility.

If you don't know how a pregnancy test works, basically it detects the hormone <u>Human Chorionic Gonadotropin</u> (hCG) in a woman's urine. hCG is secreted by a developing placenta after a fertilized egg implants in the uterine lining. Therefore, it's a red flag for conception. This hormone rises in concentration during gestational growth, so it is also measured over time to ensure the fetus is continuing to develop.

Before going to bed, I warn Tigger and Puck that this may be it. It's the end to their rule of our peaceful household. They'll have a little more than nine months to get ready for a crying baby to completely abolish life as they know it. Then I pat my stomach and tell our baby girl or boy, "I can't wait to meet you." I am so excited that I can't imagine falling asleep, but the dreams finally come.

HOPE

I've been feeling a little like a rat in a cage, not knowing if pushing the button will give me a shock or a food pellet. So far, I haven't gotten any food pellets no matter how many times I've pushed the button.

I'd convinced Michelle that maybe just having sex when it was time wasn't enough. So this past month, we ramped up the sex. We went at it like rabbits. Or at least 30-year-old rabbits with full time jobs, responsibilities and major distractions like *Sports Center* and *Gray's Anatomy*. I felt really good about it. I felt like this was it.

On our walk, we talked about the child that might be, about the process and even about writing this book. My job, my goal, is always the same—to make her laugh and to keep the thread of hope alive.

Michelle is late after eight months of trying. Is this the month? I'm so full of anticipation I begin to read a book about embryo development. The baby would be the size of a pinhead right now, but will be growing very fast. I can only wait and hope.

LESSON 12: IMAGINE THE POSITIVE AND STAY IN THE MOMENT.

ALMOST

I wake up at 2:00 a.m. with cramps. It feels like my ovaries are being twisted in a knot. I groan like a dying llama. I stumble to the bathroom for the pregnancy test I was saving for tomorrow and read the instructions on the box through a bleary gaze.

What happened to pink (or was it blue) means pregnant? Why don't they just use red and green like a stoplight?

This one makes you compare two horizontal lines. If both lines look the same—jackpot. If the test line is lighter or the second line doesn't show up at all, it's back to the drawing board.

Note to self—buy the more expensive version next time that says the words "Pregnant" or "Not Pregnant" right on the stick. I want to kick myself for being a cheap ass.

I wait three minutes, but the second line never appears. Maybe I need to wait longer? Five minutes later, with one lonely test line still looking for its pair, I give up. This never would have happened with the stoplight pregnancy test. I slump back to bed and break down in tears. I thought this was finally it. It's the middle of the night, but I need my husband to console me. I feel the need to share my sadness. I feel the need to share my sadness. I count deer instead and finally fall back to sleep an hour later.

My period is light and I'm still nauseous four days later, so I break down and call the doctor's office. The nurse suggests I go in for a blood test just in case I'm pregnant.

At the lab, I wonder how often people come in for a pregnancy test but don't want to be pregnant. I wonder what's going through the head of the college girl taking my blood. It's probably far off from what I'm thinking about, which is babies, babies, babies. She says the results will be ready by the afternoon and I smile and say, "Wish me luck!"

But there is no luck to be had this time. A call comes in and the nurse delivers the three words I expect, but don't want to hear—"You're not pregnant."

PART II

DESPERATELY SEEKING ASSISTANCE

A SEARCH FOR THE MISSING INGREDIENT

It's been ten cycles without success. How hard can this be? It feels like I'd have a better chance of winning the lottery by now. Doesn't it only take one good egg and one strong swimming sperm with a sense of direction (does it even need that?) to make it happen? Aren't these little buggers hardwired to find the egg?

We start to wonder if there is a missing ingredient. I'm 30, Chris is 34 and unless the Fountain of Youth is discovered some time soon, our chances of getting pregnant decrease with each passing month. It's time to find out more. Since we haven't hit a year of trying yet, I decide to talk to my OB/GYN first. I'm ovulating regularly so she suggests checking my <u>progesterone</u> level after ovulation next, especially since my cycles are on the shorter end of the spectrum (24 days versus an average of 28).

According to the test, my progesterone levels are just fine. Well, that's good news I guess. Two check marks down, a dozen more to go.

The next step is to make sure the egg and sperm are getting to the right place. That's where the Hysterosalpingogram (HSG) test comes in. It's an x-ray to make sure your fallopian tubes aren't blocked and to check for other uterine abnormalities.

Just before my sister got pregnant with her first child, she had this test done. She warned me that the cramping could be a little overwhelming and wanted to be there to offer support and drive me home. Since Chris will be out of town, she volunteers to drive in from San Antonio to go to the test with me. Always the big sister—looking out for me.

Laura and I are about four years apart, so we never had much to fight over. But then, we never had much in common either, until we'd grown up.

Should I bother checking if my non-fertility covering insurance will pay for this test? The answer is most likely no, so I don't even make the call.

A week later, Laura and I arrive at the Austin Radiological Association, located in a strip mall between a Gold's Gym and a Bingo warehouse. Maybe we can win a round of Bingo while we wait for the test results. I sign in and then sit patiently in the waiting room, catching up with Laura while sneaking in a little kid watching—a habit of mine these days. A little boy wipes his bright green booger onto his younger sister's hair. He's a smart one though—he looks up at his mom first to make sure she isn't watching. That's the kind of kid I want.

I think of my mom and smile, imagining the terrified expression she'd have watching the germs spread. There was no such thing as a five second rule in my house. If you dropped something on the floor, that was it. In fact, if something even looked at the floor, it was thrown away immediately. There was no sharing off of a plate anywhere near where your fork had touched. And of course, drink sharing was unthinkable. The one time she caught my sister drinking out of the milk carton, she gasped and nearly passed out in horror.

Chris calls my mom "Dr. Howell," because she's constantly reading up on the latest medical research pertaining to anything and everything—especially regarding the ailments of our family. She's also relentless once you tell her about any kind of pain. I made the mistake of mentioning Chris' shoulder injury in the early days of our dating and every time she saw Chris she asked him about it—even years later after he'd had surgery and his shoulder had healed.

My mom also needs to be stressed about something at all times, so worrying about other people helps to fill the gaps when there's nothing for her to worry about.

My dad is one of those happy people who always has a smile on his face and twinkle in his eye. His response to, "How are you?" is "Fantastic!" or "Stupendous!" He's also the most patient, laid-back member of our family. I can remember him raising his voice two times in my childhood. Both times, Laura had pushed him over the edge. Because of her work on them, I was the angel daughter who could do no wrong. Thank you big sis!

I'm jerked back to the present by the sound of my name being called. The receptionist leads me back to the changing area where I am greeted by the unflattering gown. Who makes these things? And why do they design them so your butt hangs out the back? There must be a better way. I wonder if someone could build a successful company around fashionable hospital gowns. I guess they'd only sell to the very posh clinics and private hospitals. Still, there might be a good business idea in there somewhere.

We're whisked down into a fluorescently lit examination room by a living, breathing Barbie doll. Her cohort, a shorter blond with a kind face, talks me through the entire process step by step.

She explains: "A speculum will be inserted to make room for a catheter pushed into your cervix that injects a dye through your uterus and fallopian tubes. The die can reveal problems with the tubes, such as an abnormal structure or a blockage that would prevent an egg from reaching the uterus. A clear path of dye means a clear path for the egg to get to the uterus. The test also helps to determine the shape and overall health of the uterus."

Got it. The process is sounding awfully similar to a plumber unclogging a drain.

Barbie asks Laura to leave the room to avoid radiation from the x-ray machine. I'm on my own. I take a deep breath.

The speculum is cold steel and needless to say, uncomfortable, but I grit my teeth, knowing that won't be the worst of it. The technician warns me that I'll feel pressure once she reaches the cervix. Yup—there's definitely some pressure there followed by a sharp pain. But yet again, not the worst part. Then she inflates a balloon inside the catheter to prevent the dye from leaking out of my uterus. Now I have a beach ball inside my vagina.

Wham. There it is. The cramps come fast and violent, eating away at my insides. I writhe on the table in pain. Was that groan out loud? I grip the side of the table so fiercely all the blood rushes from my fingertips. I should have gone to play Bingo instead.

I watch on the screen as Barbie has me adjust my position and the other tech moves the x-ray machine around for pictures. The dye snakes through my tubes without a hitch and the blondes are all smiles, confirming that everything looks good. Tubes clear? Check. Uterus clear? Check.

Then I wonder. Do I really want everything to look good? I guess I do, but still, it would have been nice to have an AHA MOMENT that explained why I hadn't gotten pregnant yet.

Barbie says, "I bet you'll be pregnant in two months." That's the other benefit of this test. Sometimes it increases your chances of getting pregnant, since the tubes are now flushed out. Laura was pregnant a month after her HSG test, so there might be some truth to the pitch. Who knew some dye and a beach ball could do such good work?

Once the photo shoot of my ovaries is done, the balloon is deflated and the catheter and speculum are removed. AAHHHHH. Immediate relief. And that is it. The dye rushes out of me as I sit up and I head to the bathroom to clean up and change.

Barbie lets me know that the x-ray technician will review the films and provide an official report to my doctor, and that my doctor will then follow up with me. I leave the clinic feeling good. No aha moment, but a problem with my tubes would definitely mean advanced fertility treatments, which I'm not necessarily ready for yet. Though that could certainly get us to our goal faster.

THE STATISTICS

Statistics mean everything and nothing at the same time. I use them as a guide and I would advise you to as well. Your doctor certainly will be using them. For example, most doctors will tell you not to seek any type of fertility testing or treatment until after you have been trying for a year without success—unless there is a known issue or the couple is 35 or older. That's because the statistics show most couples will conceive on their own in that time period.

The statistics say that if there isn't a problem, Michelle should be pregnant by now. We've been trying for far too long to not have any success.

Many people don't want to know they have a problem. I swim against the current on that one. I want to understand the problem and I want to know how to fix it. I am by nature a problem solver, and in this case, I want the problem to be me, because if it is, it should be easy to fix. As long as I have a few healthy sperm floating around in there, then all else can be worked out.

But if we can't figure out the why, the bottom line statistically isn't that bad. For a majority of couples with fertility issues, in vitro fertilization (IVF) success rates are very high. The percentages vary by clinic, issue and age, but on average, 30% of couples will conceive on their first IVF try, around 40% on their second, and more than 60% will have conceived by their third IVF cycle. Nearly two in three couples.

Essentially, we'll pay someone around $12,000 per IVF cycle to grab my sperm and my wife's eggs and join them together to dance in the warmth of a petri dish. Three or five days later, the best one or two embryos will be reinserted into Michelle's uterus via a mini "turkey baster" and hopefully one attaches to the uterine lining resulting in a pregnancy. Think of it as the "meet cute" in a romantic comedy. That's Hollywood speak for the unique way love interests first meet in a movie. But instead of Matthew McConaughey knocking over Kate Hudson, it's my sperm punching its way into Michelle's egg.

Twelve thousand dollars to get what I worried might happen on a drunken, careless night in college. Clearly the tables have turned.

Two in three is not a certainty, but there is one thing for certain. I am determined to have a sense of humor about this journey. To make it an adventure. After all, none of this may work out at all, and Michelle and I could be stuck with a gaping hole where we wanted a child to be.

When we discuss the possibility of never having children, we agree we'll travel, spoil our nieces and enjoy life to the fullest. But I know now that something will be missing, and this will be tough to get over. So my job is to ease us through this. I love her and can't imagine life without a happy, healthy Michelle.

But I'm getting a little ahead of myself. We're not ready for IVF quite yet. Until then, I'm following the statistics and looking for answers that will get a healthy egg and sperm together to form a baby.

LESSON 13: NUMBERS TELL ONLY PART OF THE TRUTH.

THE FIRST SIGN OF A PROBLEM

Based on the technicians' reactions, I'd assumed the HSG report would be positive. (You would think these people wouldn't toy with my emotions like that.) But a few days after the HSG test, I get a call from my OB, who says, "I'd like you to go in for another test. One of the x-rays showed what looked like a fibroid."

I had no idea what a <u>uterine fibroid</u> was at the time. It sounded like a nutritional line item on the back of a protein bar that I always glossed over. Don't have enough fibroid in your diet? Eat one of these protein bars that taste like tree bark.

Fibroid tumors are solid masses made of fibrous tissue (hence the name) typically found in the uterus. Uterine fibroids range in size, but can grow to be as big as a grapefruit.

In case you are (a) in the medical field and know all about fibroids, (b) one of those people who knows something about everything, (c) don't need any details about fibroids, (d) so fascinated with our story that you can't wait to continue, and/or (e) still thinking fibroids are an ingredient in protein bars, then we won't go into any more details here. If you want to know more about fibroids, head to the back of the book to Appendix B and then return here when you're ready. You wouldn't want to miss anything.

Still here or just coming back? Okay then. Onward.

My OB explains that this next test is easy—"just an ultrasound." In an <u>ultrasound</u>, high-pitched sound waves travel from a handheld instrument placed either on the abdomen or inside the vagina. These sound waves bounce off of internal organs to create a picture on a monitor. Think of those green-screen SONAR monitors that submarine captains use in movies, only the blinking dot approaching is a fibroid rather than a giant octopus or Godzilla. Well who knows, maybe there is an octopus in my uterus. I've already had a beach ball in there and been warned of a possible grapefruit, so nothing is out of the realm of possibility.

I am told the process is relatively painless. However,

the nurse failed to mention the discomfort I am bound to feel with a bladder ready to burst, due to the two bottles of water I'd been instructed to drink within an hour of my appointment (something about the water helping to move organs out of the way for a clearer picture of my uterus).

I thought getting the water down was the hard part. Keeping it in is harder. I feel like I'm about to explode and they haven't even called me back yet. I tell myself not to think about water. Or rain. Or waterfalls. Or anything that could let loose Niagara Falls. Still, I have visions of draining my bladder right on this lumpy chair. I look down to see if the chairs are already stained. Maybe my mess will just blend in. I scan the room for a target to dump the blame on. Darn. Where are the potty training toddlers when you need one?

Ten minutes later, I'm in my favorite hospital garb and unfortunately my butt is still swaying in the breeze of the air conditioning. But this examination room is a stark contrast to the fluorescent HSG room. It's as dark as a dance club and it takes my eyes several seconds to adjust to see my hands. Luckily, it's also very quiet, because any sound related to water would definitely make me pee at this point. If Chris were in this situation, he probably would have peed in the office plant 20 minutes ago.

My mind wanders to a safe place. I'm walking through Disney World, through the gates, down Main Street, right into Tommorowland and so on and so on...

My technician is the equivalent of a cardboard

cutout with the personality of a brick wall. She is robotic, devoid of any expression, and she remains that way throughout the test. The Terminator would have brought more colorful personality to the procedure.

There's no play-by-play on what to expect this time—she just dives right in, placing an ultrasound wand on my stomach. The monitor is facing away from me. I wonder if that's protocol or power trip? I ask her, "Can you see the fibroid?" but she actually grunts in response and I can't tell if the grunt indicates a yes or no. Gosh, what is wrong with this lady? Maybe she has a grapefruit in her uterus?

I now fully appreciate how great my last technicians were. I suppose they figure the most personable techs should cover the HSG test, which is stressful and a little painful, and the least personable ones end up in the shadowy ultrasound rooms where they aren't supposed to tell you anything anyway.

Is that water dripping in a sink? Drip, drip, drip. The faint sound calls out to my bladder, urging me to just let go. I think I just felt a little pee seep out.

The robot posing as a woman has me roll around in different positions like a ballerina. She's squinting at the screen—does she see an octopus? Then she finally speaks. "I want to do another test—this one will be vaginal—but you can get up and relieve your bladder first."

Is that good or bad? I finally get to pee, but I still don't have any answers.

I hobble down to the bathroom, clenching my

thighs together so I don't dribble pee onto the floor. It takes what seems like at least five minutes to purge the two bottles of water.

Not knowing what to expect, I'm hesitant to leave the safety of the bathroom. Now that I don't have to pee anymore, I could just stay in here for a while and chill. But I suppose she'd search me out sooner or later. I sigh, flip off the bathroom light and trudge back to the table.

The rest of the test isn't as bad as I'd imagined. She warns me I need a <u>vaginal ultrasound</u> and then inserts a lubricated wand up there, wiggles it around a bit, strikes a few keys on the computer keyboard (snapping pictures? Facebooking?), and after a few minutes, she's finished.

"So, when will I find out the results?" I ask.

"Your doctor will give you a call," she replies.

Very insightful. Thank you so much for your caring demeanor and helpful response.

I sit up and shake her, yelling, "TELL ME! TELL ME!"

I must not know my own strength because her robot head falls off and drops to the floor with a loud crash. I consider trying to get her head back on, but she looks like C3PO in the Cloud City. There are so many wires I give up and flee.

My OB calls me two days later to say everything looks fine. No sign of a fibroid. Another check mark.

Ovulating? Check. Enough progesterone? Check.

Fallopian Tubes and Uterus fine? Check. No fibroids messing up my fertility? Check. Those were all the tests on my OB's list, so now it's Chris' turn.

TESTING THE SWIMMERS

I'm shuffling around the house, tired and plagued with allergies. My nose is running, I'm sneezing and I feel like I've been hit by a giant purple pollen tree out of a Dr. Seuss book.

Michelle has already started some fertility testing, and so far, none of them have provided any answers. So far, so good. Or is it? We still know nothing. And without knowing, there really isn't a way to actively solve the problem. So I fester in my free flowing body fluids.

It's my turn to be tested tomorrow and I can't imagine going in feeling like this. I head into the kitchen to drink some tea to try and clear up my sinuses. I dunk the tea bag into the piping hot water. Color seeps into the water, darkening the liquid until it's brown and opaque.

Michelle walks in; she's still stressed about this whole process but seems cheerful this morning. She looks at me, glances into the glass. I tip it toward my lips, and she claws at the cup before I can take a sip. I think she is playing and I feign like I am going to release it, but then I try to drink it again. She grabs it harder and I laugh.

"You can't have caffeine anymore," she says.

I grunt, not understanding.

"Caffeine can lower your sperm count."

I still want something hot to drink.

Speaking of sperm counts, that is my test tomorrow.

I want to make myself feel better, so I head back to the cabinet and snag the hot chocolate. Michelle shakes her head, no.

"That has caffeine in it too."

I shoot her a dirty look.

"Better safe than sorry."

I want to melt into the floor.

***

The next morning, Michelle is prodding me to hurry so I won't be late. I counter that it is not likely that they'll start without me. Then I ask her, "Do you think they help?"

She laughs. "I doubt it. But you can ask." Then she mumbles, "It'll probably be some burly man or a woman the size of a refrigerator."

On my way, I can't help but think that it is strange that everyone at the office will know exactly what I am doing. I feel like a teenage boy who locks himself away in the bathroom for an hour to "experiment."

I practice my greeting. "Hello—I'm here to jack off

into a cup."

It's a small office, a vague description on the door, Urologist. I walk into the lobby, about fifteen old plastic chairs, half filled with gray-haired old men. At the far end behind a glass window is a reception booth with a cute blond already eyeing me curiously. She's not the size of a refrigerator and she is certainly not a burly man.

I tell her my name and she smiles and raises her eyebrows. I get the feeling that all the other patients in the lobby didn't get that greeting—it's reserved for those making special donations.

She tells me to sign in and then hold tight for a minute. I sit down and grab a magazine. No pornos out here—I guess they save those for the rooms.

After a few minutes of pretending to read, the woman from the desk comes through the door dangling a key. She smiles and asks me to follow her. This reminds me of the way I would imagine checking into a seedy hotel.

We make small talk as we walk down the hallway, up a back staircase and then past a few doors. She uses the key on an unmarked door.

She waves me into the room—a "Comfort Inn" cheap hotel room with a recliner in place of a bed—and then follows me in. A wave of nervousness ripples through my body. Is she staying? I was joking when I asked about assistance—this is embarrassing enough as it is.

She asks me if I am comfortable. I nod nervously; I can feel my skin beginning to sweat. She gives me a tour of the place, as if I'm buying a new home. She points out a chair, a sink, several sets of drawers, and the all-important specimen cup where the sperm will go. She opens a drawer with lubrication and another drawer chock full of nudie magazines. She holds a couple up to show me that they are there, and I suspect to assure me it's okay to use them—I'm not a fifteen-year-old anymore. Even in this situation, there is something incredibly sexy about a woman holding a magazine with a nude woman on the cover.

The receptionist glances at me with a wide smirk, suggesting she knows the deed I am about to perform. She tells me to flip a switch when I am done and leave the cup on the table. The lab next door will pick up the sample. Now that she mentions it, I can hear people chattering in the room next door. It's the lab, and I imagine that there is a centrifuge and test tubes and men in white coats, but I am losing my focus. She is leaving, and I need to pay attention. She says goodbye and closes the door behind her. I can hear it lock as it shuts.

I now feel very alone and the voices next door seem too close. But I sigh, resigned to the fact that I have a job to do.

LESSON 14: I AM NO LONGER JUST ALONG FOR THE RIDE.

ANOTHER CHECK MARK

My OB/GYN recommended a <u>semen analysis</u> for Chris as the last step before seeing a fertility specialist.

I can't speak to much of this process, except to say that Chris thought I should owe him a lot for going through it. Finding out there's a required two to four day abstinence makes him even grumpier. He needs to get over it. I've had a beach ball and fairy godmother's wand shoved up my vagina for our future child.

The results are back within a week and the nurse runs through the results over the phone, which I frantically copy down. She suggests that even though some of Chris' numbers are a little lower than average, everything looks okay. I ask for a copy of the report since I don't understand any of the details she's just told me (other than the fact that I'm the reason we're not pregnant yet). I look at my notes scratched onto the back of an envelope. What's Motility? Viscosity? Morphology? It's back to the Internet to do some research. Want to know more? See Appendix C for a list of semen analysis definitions.

After comparing Chris' numbers to what is considered "average," I'm not sure where that leaves us. I call my OB/GYN and she suggests that some of Chris' numbers—count and motility especially—are concerning. She suggests that he check with an expert.

The nurse had made it seem like while a couple numbers were borderline, they should not be an issue. Now my OB is indicating otherwise. What's the real story? Are his numbers a problem or not? Could this really be the reason I'm not pregnant yet? I'm skeptical, but it is the first fertility test we haven't been able to put a definitive check mark next to.

Chris claims he's glad he could be the problem. He figures that will make me feel better if we can't ever have children—that I won't be able to blame myself. He's right. But I'm not sure I want to be able to blame him either.

A week later, Chris has me come with him to see the sperm specialist. (Who would want to look at sperm all day? Or penises?) Chris is the youngest male in the waiting room by at least 30 years. The doctor says Chris' latest batch of numbers looks fine and shouldn't prevent us from getting pregnant. But there could be an anatomical reason for our troubles. So he has Chris drop his boxers. It is a very interesting experience being on the other end—watching Chris be examined. But it's not like he had to put his feet in stirrups like women do. Not even close.

Everything checked out fine anatomically. The problem, whatever it is, lies with me. It is finally time to consult with the fertility experts.

SO FAR

I've been commiserating with a friend of mine, who just started the fertility rigmarole with his wife. I tell him what to expect when he has to give his sample at the office.

He calls me the morning of. "It's 9:00 a.m. I'm smoking a cigar and walking the dog."

A few weeks later his numbers come back and they aren't so good. His wife is quick to point out that he celebrated prematurely—he should have waited to smoke the cigar after he got the results. Ouch! But hey, they're both laughing about it and getting through it.

Still, I am going to have to remember to be even nicer to Michelle.

What began in my mind as one month of great sex has now been stretched and contorted into something else entirely. And unfortunately, it is not something out of Kama Sutra. I blame the Miller Curse.

I've had some good sex sure, but I've also had to "excite" myself in a doctor's office while people were listening. I've dropped my shorts and had a doctor examine my junk with my wife watching. And I've accomplished nothing. We have no answer; we are no closer. It feels like darkness is descending and I need a match, a burning ember, to see the forest through the trees.

LESSON 15: WE ARE CLUELESS.

THE CONTINUED SEARCH

It has now been a year. Fourteen cycles have come and gone. We are now officially branded with the infertility label with no answer as to why.

When people have no idea you've been trying to get pregnant, they say a lot of annoying things that get under your skin. "Why don't you two have any kids yet?" "You'd make great parents." "What are you waiting for?" Or my all-time favorite—"Don't you want a family?"

First, I have a family, whether I'm able to bare children or not. Second, yes I do want children very much, which is why I've been going in for uncomfortable doctor visits and tests. I hear the thoughts in my head as I write and realize little whispers of bitterness have begun gnawing at my brain.

Pregnant women can be pretty batty, especially

those who had no problems conceiving. One friend said (while rolling her eyes), "I expected to get pregnant after the first month, but it actually took us two tries. I was so worried!" She popped open a bottle of wine and began to pour. I wanted to pop her head off like that wine cork.

One of my friends, who is in the same boat fertility-wise, almost slapped a girl in her book club when she said, "I was so depressed—it took us FIVE MONTHS to get pregnant!" Really? Five whole months? That must have been really tough. How did you survive?

Even those who know Chris and I are trying say things that are pretty annoying. "I don't know how you do it. I'd be going crazy by now." Or, "You just need to stop stressing about it, go on a vacation and eat some ice cream." Is that all we need to do? A vacation and ice cream and we'll be all set? Good to know! I'm glad that doesn't apply to everyone, because we'd have a lot of knocked up teenagers after Spring Break every year.

I do feel like I've had a pretty healthy attitude up to this point, mostly because I know there are so many fertility treatment options these days. I'm confident that Chris and I will find a way to have children. That said, I'm close to my breaking point and the next clueless comment might catapult me over the edge.

At least we're progressing to the next step. The fertility clinic with the most experience in Austin is not on our current insurance, not that our insurance covers anything related to fertility anyway. The first consultation alone is $275. Chris and I actually discuss moving to Boston and finding jobs there so all these fertility bills would be covered. Delusions of grandeur. Massachusetts is one of only a few states where fertility coverage is mandatory for insurance providers. In Texas, insurance companies must offer fertility coverage, but the difference in monthly premiums is so high (25%+) that very few companies elect to choose this coverage for their employees.

I schedule the first available appointment—four days before Christmas—with the clinic's most experienced doctor. Maybe we'll luck out and get pregnant on our own so I can happily call to cancel that appointment. A quiet victory, and money saver. That's what happened to my sister with her first pregnancy.

***

But alas, that's not to be. November and half of December fly by without success and before we know it, it's time for our first fertility visit. I've barely finished scribbling my name in the log when the receptionist asks for my credit card.

Chris and I almost went to medical school back in the day and I find myself pondering that if we returned to school now and wanted to make a ton of money, fertility seems like a winner of a specialty. Relatively happy patients and most of them rack up their bills on credit cards. I'm so lost in thought that I don't notice the receptionist holding out my card.

The office reminds me of an expensive hotel lobby, with posh couches, leather chairs, dark wood coffee tables and a fish tank covering one wall. It's a subtle reminder that I am paying for this. There is a reception desk that looks like a business office, with the door to the doctor's office on one side and a secure entrance on the other. I sink down into an empty couch and watch the fish for a while. Then I furtively peak at the other patients.

There is only one woman and a couple waiting. I wonder what their stories are. The woman farthest from me appears to be about my age. She's dressed in a bank teller navy suit and the rock on her finger screams money. She can probably buy the practice so she doesn't have to wait in line. By the way she flips patiently through her magazine, I'd guess she's been in this waiting room many times.

The couple is whispering sweet nothings and laughing with each other on the couch across from mine. They also look to be in their early thirties. Do they know what their issue is or are they in the dark like we are? Are they at the beginning stages or have they been through the ropes with multiple in vitro attempts to no avail? By their easygoing manner, they might even be pregnant. Could be, they're awaiting their first heartbeat sonogram.

My OB's office was supposed to have sent all of our files over, but I brought Chris' numbers (his sperm counts sounds like lottery numbers at this point) along with a pad of paper filled with questions.

Chris arrives just as they're calling my name and we're escorted to Dr. Vaughn's office. I warm up to our doctor after just a few minutes. He's Santa Clause without the snowy beard and fat tummy. His eyes crease when he smiles and he has a soothing voice that says, "I know what you're going through," even though he may not really know what it's like to be on this side of the desk. We chose Dr. Vaughn because he has the most experience of any of the fertility doctors in Austin and every review was glowing.

I'd already done a lot of research about the clinic online. But I brought a list of questions that I was ready to fire off.

Question 1—What do you recommend next after the steps we've already checked off our list (with the ovulation, progesterone and HSG tests all normal)?

He is direct. "You have two options. You can continue to try to figure out what the problem is. In that case, we'll do some additional tests like a blood test to measure your FSH and a laparoscopy and hysteroscopy to make sure you don't have endometriosis. Or you can go straight into fertility treatments, which often solve the problem whatever the issue is."

Dr. Vaughn adds that typically, diagnostic tests are covered by insurance, while fertility treatments are not, so that could impact the decision.

Question 2—What type of treatment do you usually

try first?

"If we go the testing route, it will depend on what I find after the FSH test and laparoscopy. If we skip the tests, then <u>Clomid</u> is usually step one, or you can skip right to <u>injectables</u> or IVF. It depends on your timetable."

Question 3—Are you comfortable with us doing our own research and suggesting a particular treatment?

"Absolutely."

I look back down at my question list and think he's covered everything I need to know for now.

MEETING DR. VAUGHN

Three things strike me about my first visit to the Texas Fertility Clinic.

First, there are swarms of young, happy, attractive women working in this office. There are always ten or more nurses and office staff there to support the three doctors in the practice.

Second, there is a very colorful fish tank. I have a feeling that I'm going to become good friends with these fish.

Third, we've picked the right doctor.

The first thing Dr. Vaughn asks about is our sex life. It strikes me as odd, not that he asks, but that this seems so natural. How things can change in so little time. I'm talking to a complete stranger about my sex life in front of my wife and there is absolutely no alcohol involved.

He recommends we stop the scheduling and just go back to having sex when we want to. Hell Yeah! I love this guy.

The weight on my shoulders is lifted. His concern is not just about us getting pregnant, but also our general well being. The key is that he's been here before. Maybe not personally. But he's guided couples through this process time and time again.

LESSON 16: FIND A GREAT DOCTOR. IT'S ONE OF THE ONLY THINGS YOU CAN CONTROL.

THE FIRST MISSING CHECK MARK

Chris and I are leaning toward the testing route before diving into fertility treatments. Chris' company is changing insurance policies in a few months and because the fertility clinic doesn't accept our current insurance, but will take the new one, we decide to wait until then.

More waiting.

More sex.

More disappointment.

While we're in limbo, I get a call from Dr. Vaughn. He informs me that they recently received the results of my HSG and ultrasound tests and he had his own sonogram technician review them and then reviewed them himself. They DID see a fibroid and that may be causing a problem.

One minute I'm happily shopping for shoes, and the next minute I'm told I have a fibroid. Could this be what's causing our infertility? I think it is safe to assume my fibroid is pretty small (not the size of a grapefruit), or the OB's office would surely have seen it, right?

Dr. Vaughn tells me if I decide on a laparoscopy to check for endometriosis, there's a chance he'll be able to remove the fibroid at the same time. However, if the fibroid is inside the uterine lining, that would require a different, more intense surgical procedure. Please be the former.

Houston, we have a problem.

I call Chris to break the news. Then I walk out of the store empty handed. Goodbye, pretty silver shoes. I can't afford you anymore—I have an insurance deductible to pay for.

THINGS ARE NOT GOING ACCORDING TO PLAN

Chris and I decide to go ahead with a <u>laparoscopy</u> and <u>hysteroscopy</u> (these are done at the same time) to make sure there isn't endometrial tissue in abnormal locations preventing me from getting pregnant. The benefit of this procedure is that, if they do find endometriosis, they can often clear out the tissue while you're under the knife. They may be able to remove my fibroid as well.

Wasn't all this supposed to be easy? The plan was: Step #1—Meet the love of your life. Step #2—Get married. Step #3—Have kids. Step #4—Watch them grow up. Step #5—Retire. Step #6—Play with grand-kids at vacation house somewhere sunny.

That doesn't seem like so much to ask, does it?

Now I'm scheduling a surgery where a doctor will scrape the insides of my uterus and pull out a fibroid (hopefully!) just to try to complete step #3.

***

A few days before my surgery, I go in for a blood test to measure my <u>FSH</u> and <u>estradiol</u> numbers. The amount of the follicle stimulating hormone (FSH) in your blood is important because FSH stimulates <u>follicle</u> growth in the ovaries. Without FSH, the eggs won't mature and ovulation will not occur. A high FSH number can also indicate <u>premature ovarian failure</u> or a slowdown in ovarian egg reserve, which happens to most women as they head toward menopause, but for some unlucky ones, this can happen much younger. An FSH result over 10 indicates timing may be a concern. In that case, Dr. Vaughn recommends being a little more aggressive with fertility treatments.

They test my estradiol at the same time because if this figure is too high (>50), that could mask a problem with the FSH test results, meaning a number under 10 might not really mean it's under 10.

My results come back showing an FSH of 8 but an estradiol of 75.

However, I might have screwed up the test results, because I'd already taken one hormone pill for the laparoscopy procedure.

Oops.

Dr. Vaughn suggests I repeat the test after the surgery.

WHO KNEW FISHBOWLS COULD BE DANGEROUS?

When I was eight years old, my best friend Christie and I were playing at the edge of the lake behind my house. It was tadpole season and we thought it would be fun to catch a few. So I had the brilliant idea of using my glass fishbowl to store the tadpoles after we caught them. I retrieved the fish tomb from the garage where it was condemned to collect dust after my first (and last) goldfish died. Poor little Princess Orangina.

I skipped across my backyard and down to the lake with net and bowl in hand, where Christie was desperately trying to catch tadpoles with her hands. I handed her the net, filled the fishbowl with lake water and then placed it on the sandbags to await its quarry. I wanted to raise my arms to the sky in triumph over my great idea. That's when things went awry.

The shoddy fishbowl shattered on impact against the sandbags and while I was fretting about how much trouble I was going to be in for breaking a useless $5 fishbowl, a shard of glass the size of a small plate slipped down into the two-inch deep water and sliced open my big toe.

I don't remember feeling any pain then, but the sight of the water growing dark red induced panic. I limped up to the house, leaving a trail of blood, to wake my parents from their Saturday afternoon nap. That was my second mistake, because I would learn later that my hobble through the thick grass was probably what snapped the tendon in my toe.

I remember perching on the kitchen counter while my dad doctored the bubbling wound and my mom made some calls. Christie looked on in horror, waiting for her parents to come pick her up.

This would not be the last time Christie saw me in a medical crisis. A few years later when visiting her family in Maine, I would drive my one-dollar bike (just purchased at the town fair) down a very steep street, then panic, black out, and zoom off the deck and plunge into the harbor. It was low tide and I plummeted like a sack of potatoes ten feet down onto the jagged, barnacled ocean rocks. I was moved to a stretcher and rushed by speedboat to a Portland hospital, and fortunately emerged from the wreckage with only a few scrapes and bruises. If you ever find yourself in Peaks Island, Maine, you can ask one of the locals. My story is quite famous there.

I was accident-prone as a kid, if you couldn't tell.

Back to the fishbowl story. This was a bigger issue than scrapes and bruises (as evidenced by the pool of blood splayed on the kitchen floor), so my parents soon rushed me to the emergency room. My mother's best friend since childhood is married to a plastic surgeon and he agreed to handle the procedure.

All I remember before the surgery is making my parents promise they would be there when I woke up. My parents never broke their promises, so I was confident heading into the operating room that I would see their faces right after the surgery.

Strike one in the promise category. My mom and dad weren't waiting for me in the recovery room and the nurses were stuck trying to calm a screaming eight-year-old. I flailed my arms like a fish to let the nurses know how I felt about this, the IV tube flying through the air.

My parents had been assured I would be passed out for at least an hour after the surgery. Ergo, they wandered off to the cafeteria. Meanwhile, I woke up from the anesthesia just as they were rolling me into the recovery room. It took me months to forgive my parents.

So jump forward nearly twenty-five years later to my next surgery (thankfully I was only accident-prone as a child). Dr. Vaughn promises me that the laparoscopy will be quick and easy—a thirty minute procedure, an hour in the recovery room and a day of rest at home and I'll be back to my old self. And Chris has promised to be there when I wake up. All of these promises echo my last experience. I'm deeply skeptical.

MICHELLE'S FIRST FERTILITY SURGERY

I lie in bed thinking about Michelle's surgery tomorrow. I worry that I will leave something unsaid. I fall asleep thinking of everything that I should tell her, just in case.

Four o'clock rolls around and the alarm rattles me out of my slumber. I feel sick to my stomach. I am groggy and my brain is running at half speed. But I can't feel sorry for myself, as Michelle is the one going under the knife.

She is double checking everything. Her bag, her purse, the instructions, the map. She's blabbering on about something.

"Do you think I can brush my teeth? I might swallow some water."

"Hmmm," is my answer.

But then I remember the important thing. "I love you."

She stops, looks into my eyes and smiles.

"A LOT," I add.

LESSON 17: REMEMBER HOW MUCH YOU LOVE EACH OTHER. IF YOU DIDN'T, YOU SURE AS HELL WOULDN'T BE READING THIS.

MORE HOSPITAL GOWNS

We are told to arrive at the outpatient clinic before the sun rises. Chris circles the place four times, lost in the dark night. I'm in the process of looking at the directions as we zoom past it. Ah—now I see how this map works. It helps to have it facing the right direction.

After signing paper after paper warning me about the risks of the surgery (the word death comes up at least three times), I settle in and watch an infomercial about face powder through half-open eyes.

They call my name and it's off to the bathroom to pee in a cup. One of the forms asked if I was pregnant or trying to become pregnant, and since the latter was certainly true, I checked yes. I'm assuming they're testing to make sure I'm not pregnant, which is comforting. Oh, and of course I'm in one of the great hospital gowns again. This time there are little pink pigs smiling up at me. I consider myself young at heart, but this is ridiculous. Maybe I can design my own gown and bring it with me next time.

Once the IV is in, we're told we are just waiting for the doctor to arrive, at which time they'll put a special concoction in my IV and knock me out. Chris, always the entertainer, cracks jokes while we wait. I can also count on him to act his age, which is usually around twelve.

Dr. Vaughn arrives, the drugs are inserted into my IV and I kiss Chris goodbye, hoping that will not be the last time I have the opportunity to do so.

The bright lights on the ceiling turn to beautiful, yellow flowers and I float toward them. My rolling bed hasn't even passed through the doors before the world fades to black.

AN ACTIVE IMAGINATION

Michelle has been in surgery for a while now. Her sister has driven in from San Antonio. Laura loves her little sister and wants to be here for her. More than an hour has passed. It is supposed to be a simple procedure, and it seems like we should have received an update by now.

I'm a little choked up, recollecting the moments before they took her away. I was all laughs and jokes until they started to wheel Michelle toward the surgery room. Although I had so much to say, my throat swelled up and closed, leaving me only able to mumble.

I've never had anyone I've known go in for any surgery or even a complicated medical procedure; this is all foreign to me. Should I assume that an hour really means an hour? Or is it like a fancy restaurant where 15 minutes really means an hour. I'd imagine it has to be much more like NASA, on a tight schedule; don't they have other patients coming after this?

But if it's supposed to be an hour, do they count the time for the doctor to scrub out and come talk to us? If there is an issue, when do they tell me?

This is not a good day to have a very active imagination. I can't read anymore and my stomach hurts and I'm starting to think the worst. I stare at the chairs in the waiting room; part tired but mostly paralyzed with fear. I want an update. I need to know that she is okay. That this wasn't a big mistake.

Finally, a nurse comes out and asks for me. I am grateful for this. If there is bad news, I want to get it alone first. She takes me through the door and into the hallway and into a small conference room.

Now I am a bundle of nerves. My heart is racing as fast as Seabiscuit. This cannot possibly be normal. This seems very formal. I survey the room anxiously. Two sets of chairs facing each other. My mind furiously pieces together that this is a grieving room.

There is nothing around to throw; the paintings look to be secured to the wall. This is it. My life is about to implode.

The door swings open and I jump up. Dr. Vaughn waltzes through with a big grin etched on his face. I see no trace of regret or remorse, and he can probably see the relief on mine. I resume breathing. My eyes fill with tears. He tells me the laparoscopy went well and that Michelle is recovering. They were able to remove a bit of endometriosis, but the fibroid was embedded in the uterine wall and could not be removed.

He says congratulations—you're ready to begin. Begin fertility treatments. Begin more procedures. Begin the rest of our lives.

I shake his hand. This seems like the thing to do, and it feels like a great moment. I tell him good job and thanks.

LESSON 18: THIS IS JUST THE BEGINNING?

NOT THIS LEG!

When I come to, a nurse is sitting in a chair at the end of my bed, scribbling notes and looking after me. She asks how I'm feeling and hands me some crackers. I fall back to sleep before I can answer her.

The second time around I'm awake for good and she encourages me to get to my feet and try out my legs. Why? Did they operate on the wrong body parts? Should I have written *Not This Leg!* *on the right one and Not This Leg Either!* on the left with a Sharpie?

MICHELLE LOSES HER MIND— TEMPORARILY

I wait for Michelle in the recovery room. It's a shared room with space for up to four beds, all partitioned by curtains. The one Michelle will be in is as empty as the other three.

It's quiet except for the noise of daytime TV echoing down the halls. Then I hear a new noise. A voice—that of a nurse—and it sounds like she is coddling a child.

I see the colorful scrubs of a nurse and a hunched figure walking beside her. I realize it's Michelle taking baby steps, like a child learning to walk. Her head is tilted down, hair covering her face, her hands stretched out in front like she is reaching for something. She looks somewhere between the most fragile thing I have ever seen and a Scooby Doo villain, moaning, hunched with arms extending blindly.

The nurse guides her gently. She gets halfway to the room. Something is wrong. She stops and tilts her head awkwardly. The complexion drains from her face. I've heard the expression turning green and this it is precisely. The nurse knows she is ready to blow, and so do I.

The nurse says, "You feel nauseous?" and is already steering Michelle toward the bathroom.

Michelle has come out again and the nurse pilots her to the bed. I feel horrible for her. She's finding her way clumsily under the covers. I can't stand to let her struggle like this. I help her into bed.

Michelle asks me how the surgery went. I explain the results.

"Did he get the fibroid?" she asks.

"No." I explain that it was embedded too much in the wall.

Her chin quivers.

I tell her to sit back, relax and drink some water. Michelle drinks a few sips and then leans back. I'm trying to get her to relax and make her comfortable. She doesn't appear to be thinking clearly. She's slow, and she is never slow. This scares me a bit, but I remind myself this must be the drugs.

I ask Michelle how she feels. She says fine. I don't tell her this, but she looks like she just got back from a rave. Bloodshot eyes, frizzed hair, parched lips. I help her force down a saltine. I gobble down one myself. Yum. I don't remember them tasting this good. I think about it and realize it's probably because all the worry is gone. This is my celebration saltine.

Michelle squeezes her eyes shut for a few minutes and I hold her hand. She drifts off. I realize that the surgery being over is the end of this process for me. For me, waiting for her to come out was the hard part. She has a longer journey; she still has to heal.

Michelle's eyes open and she smiles at me.

Then she asks me, "How did the surgery go?"

I'd be worried, except that the doctor had warned us about a temporary loss of short-term memory. I laugh and tell her everything went fine.

"And did they get the fibroid?" she asks.

I can't hold it back. I erupt with boisterous laughter.

Michelle smiles and says, "I've asked you that already, haven't I?"

We go through the entire routine one more time to accommodate her goldfish memory. And then Michelle is back to normal and all is right in the world. Well, almost right.

LESSON 19: ANESTHESIA SURE CAN MESS WITH YOUR HEAD.

OR

DON'T DO DRUGS!

STILL UNLUCKY

There were two findings in the surgery. First, some minor endometriosis was found and taken care of, but my impression was that this couldn't be the main cause of my infertility. Second, as my previous luck would have predicted, the majority of the fibroid was inside the uterine lining. So if that turns out to be a problem in the future (either as a primary suspect for my infertility after we've checked everything else, or a possible cause in a future <u>miscarriage</u>), then I'll have to undergo an <u>abdominal myomectomy</u> to have the fibroid removed.

I was really hoping that damned fibroid would be gone when I woke up. I feel a little sorry for myself, stewing over my rotten luck.

THROWING CAUTION TO THE WIND

When I want something really badly, I convince myself that I'm not going to get it so that I won't be disappointed if I don't. The few times in my life where I've thrown caution to the wind and convinced myself I was going to get what I wanted, it hasn't happened and my heart fell to my stomach. So I've finally started saying, "If I can get pregnant," instead of, "When I get pregnant."

The results from my second FSH test (without any possible drug interactions this time) show a slightly elevated number of 12, so it's time to get moving before my egg production slows down even more.

<u>Clomiphene</u> (brand names Clomid, Serephone or Milophene) is usually the first step in the infertility process because it's the least expensive and invasive. You take one pill for five days during your cycle. Clomiphene is well suited for women with ovulation issues, because it increases the levels of two hormones that stimulate the ovaries and release an egg. Clomiphene works like estrogen and causes the ovaries to produce more eggs and follicles. Miracle Grow for lady parts. It is also effective in women with a <u>luteal phase</u>

defect (LPD), a condition that causes women to not produce enough progesterone, leading to issues with follicle production and/or uterine lining development.

Research shows that when lack of ovulation is the only cause of infertility, a majority of women on Clomiphene will achieve a pregnancy within six months of treatment. Since ovulation isn't my issue, Chris and I decide to skip Clomiphene and go right to gonadotropins. A baby step before in vitro. And about $3,500 a pop.

So we get on the schedule for our first injectables cycle and I'm thrilled to be moving toward a possible solution. Chris will inject shots of Gonal F into my stomach each night to (hopefully) trick my body into producing extra eggs. And then when the lead follicles are big enough (which we'll know through periodic sonograms), I'll receive another shot (hCG) that triggers the ovulation process. We will try two intra-uterine inseminations (IUIs) after the trigger shot, hoping to unite sperm and egg in the right place at the right time.

There can be moderate side effects from the drugs, but the biggest issue is we may get TOO pregnant—the stories you hear of crazy numbers of multiples (five, six, seven or even eight babies delivered at one time—hello Octomom) result from this kind of treatment gone awry. Careful monitoring should help avoid anything more than triplets, but still, the chances of getting pregnant with twins are one in five. As long as Chris and I don't end up like Jon & Kate (plus 8!), I think we will be okay.

OUR FIRST IUI

Things are finally moving forward.

Or not.

Unfortunately, our injectables plans are put on hold.

When I arrive for my day 3 sonogram, the ultrasound shows I have a cyst on one of my ovaries. I will have to wait until the cyst goes away before starting fertility treatments because the medications can react negatively with an <u>ovarian cyst</u>.

Great. I can't seem to get anything right. I haven't even started fertility treatments and my body is already uncooperative.

I picture the mass in my right ovary as an ugly, bloated head, chuckling at my bad fortune.

Dr. Vaughn suggests that we go ahead and track my ovulation and try an IUI without any drugs, just in case the problem is getting the sperm to the right place, which can happen when the semen is too thick or the pathway to the uterus is hostile.

For our IUI procedure, all we need to do is call as soon as the ovulation test turns positive, bring in the sperm-in-a-cup the next morning (which Chris is happy to be able to do from home) and then come in a couple hours later, once the sperm has been cleaned and centrifuged, to have it inserted via catheter into my cervix.

The cats aren't a huge help in the process, though they muster up great joy in pouncing around our bed at 7:00 a.m., twenty minutes before the specimen is due. Thankfully, the office is not too far away from our house. I drop off our labeled cup inside a paper bag, go back home and rest in bed, too excited to actually sleep, and then Chris and I return at 10:00 a.m. for our appointment.

Dr. Vaughn displays the IUI plunger (it looks like a giant syringe you would use to knock out an elephant) with our names on the label like it's a trophy we won.

And the award for great sperm goes to my husband, Chris Miller, encapsulated in this plunger here.

The doctor then inserts the trophy, I mean plunger, painlessly.

We wait 10 minutes before I can get up. Then we go home, hoping there's a healthy egg in there waiting to meet its healthy sperm mate.

If I have no signs of a period 14 days later, then I'll go in for a pregnancy test.

Twelve days later, my period begins.

First "official" fertility treatment down—first fertility treatment failure.

The next month Chris is scheduled to be out of town for business about the time we'd need his sperm, so we have to delay the fertility treatments once again.

At least the chances of the cyst being gone are higher now that we've given it almost two months to go away.

It's finally time to crank up my egg factory. I'm ready. We'll find out soon enough if my body is ready too.

THE TREATMENTS BEGIN

Michelle is ringing in on the other line. I'm running late for our fertility appointment and she's calling to remind me to be on time. I hang up with my client and click over to tell her I'm heading out the door.

We wait in the crowded office. A cute woman who looks like a clean-cut Helena Bonham Carter calls out Michelle's name and we head through the door together. She asks if Michelle needs to use the restroom. Not your typical question (at least not when you're a guy). And hey, she didn't ask me. I guess my needs are irrelevant at this point.

Michelle stops at the restroom and I proceed down to Room 6 at the end of the hall. Helena closes the door behind her saying she'll be back in a few minutes.

It's a simple square room, with windows on one side of the box. The shades are drawn but the room is still very bright. There is a metal chair, a stool on rollers, a table with an odd assortment of socks and a pricey instrument next to it. The place feels clinical, but comes across as warmer than most doctor's offices.

I begin, as I usually do, to investigate the instruments in the room. I jump up on the table. There are striped socks with overly loud colors sticking up from the end of the table. Pippy Longstocking has nothing on them. I inquisitively touch the socks and then yank my hand back. They don't shock me, at least not electrically. And although they are wool and itchy, it's not that either. There is metal, cold metal underneath. I take a closer look and realize that these are stirrups, and not the kind you use to ride a horse. Could be kinky, but then the wrong images of doctors with metal instruments fill my mind.

And as I lunge from the table, Michelle comes in with Helena.

"Get undressed from the waist down, use that sheet provided and sit up on the table," Helena says as she closes the door.

Michelle begins to take off her pants. I seize the moment. I unbutton my pants; pull them down to my ankles.

"Why do they need us naked from the waist down?" I ask Michelle.

Michelle laughs. At least she finds me funny. She props herself up on the table.

"Are we going to have to perform in front of them?" I ask. I can't help myself. It probably doesn't sound funny written down, but in fairness, you weren't there.

And then I pull my pants up and remember my investigation of the room. I look back at the expensive instrument next to the table. It has a panel and screen like a TV. I am proud of myself that I actually know what it is.

I tell this to Michelle.

"It's an ultrasound machine." Her tone of voice indicating there should have been a "Duh!" at the end of her sentence.

"That's not fair. You've been here before."

"It says so on the panel," she chides.

"I knew before that, I swear." I really did.

My eyes wander around the room more. I spy something that looks like a round wand. Strangely, it looks like it has a condom fastened on the end of it. My eyes bulge with excitement. I quickly glance over at Michelle who has a disapproving look on her face. If I keep it up, the wand will get more action than I do.

Just then, the door opens and I jump. Dr. Vaughn enters and asks Michelle how she's feeling.

He sees me and seems a little surprised. I wonder how many men skip out of these appointments. For me, this is an educational experience and an opportunity to support Michelle. I wouldn't miss it.

He smiles and shakes my hand. He tells us he's going to check Michelle's uterus (I guess it is like peering in a cave to make sure there are no bears) before we begin the fertility shots.

We'll be going through a "training" session later to learn more about the process, practice the shots and get our final instructions. I feel like I am training to become an MD. So this is what it would have been like.

He takes the wand and holds it up to Helena, who has come back in with him. She squirts some blue goo on it while Michelle lies down and puts her feet in the stirrups. Ready for the ride.

Images appear on the screen. I look at Michelle to see if she has any idea what we're looking at.

Pointing, Dr. Vaughn explains, "This is the cervix, and this is the uterus. When I turn to this side I am looking at the right ovary. See, it's all clear."

I think—hey—it kind of looks like a Longhorn. I remember most of the terms but I am certainly going to look up the female anatomy when I get home, because knowing how all the pieces fit together to form the Longhorn would be helpful.

"Here is the left ovary, it's all clear too." He smiles and removes the wand.

He should give the wand back to the fairy godmother. I bet she's pissed.

"It looks good. We're ready to begin."

He tells us he will give our dosages to the nurse when we leave.

Michelle gets up to dress and asks me to find her a tissue. I get her tissues and grab her clothes. I hand them both to her and give her a contemplative look.

"Does it hurt?"

"It doesn't hurt. It's just a little uncomfortable," she says.

"It seems like it would hurt."

"I'm much more worried about the shots than this. They say they can bruise and the more you get, the more painful they are each time."

Now I'm worried about the shots too. I'm the one who will be administering them.

LESSON 20: WE STILL HAVE OUR SENSE OF HUMOR.

OUR FIRST DATE

Chris and I are on our first date on the patio of Baby A's, where the food is terrible but the Everclear margaritas are pretty darn good (and so potent that they aren't supposed to serve any patron more than two). A stray black kitten comes to sit with us and share our basket of tortilla chips while Chris and I get to know each other. We talk easily and he makes me laugh so hard that a chip flies out of my nose. Very classy.

Our second stop is a movie theatre that is so packed, we are forced to sit in the very first row. For those of you who have never experienced it, sitting in the front row of an action movie after two strong margaritas is a very bad idea.

I look over at Chris, but instead of my handsome date, the Cyborg cop from Terminator 2 is sitting next to me. He rams his fist into my stomach and as I start to scream, I wake up with a jolt.

I place a hand over my stomach.

I wonder what the dream experts would say about that one.

GROW FOLLICLES, GROW

Our baseline sonogram shows we are all clear and we're finally ready for our first injectables cycle. Chris is overjoyed to be giving me the shots, which is a little unsettling. But I assume it's his love of challenges that has him pumped, not the thought of being able to jab needles into my stomach.

The drugs are supposed to arrive this morning. We leave for a walk, posting a note on the door for FedEx to **Please, Please, Please** leave the package without a signature or to ask for a neighbor's signature. I'd placed the order at 5:00 p.m. the night before, so I thought surely our package wouldn't be on the early truck.

Shows you what I know.

We return from the walk to find a note that said delivery was attempted, but a signature was required. Ugh! I frantically call FedEx to explain the situation. A few hours later, the doorbell rings and I have my medications.

That night, we read through the directions and fumble our way through the process of giving the first shot. I feel a slight prick, but no pain. We are on our way at 150 IU of Gonal F each night for the next three nights. Then we'll go back in for a sonogram to check on the progress. Grow follicles, grow!

SHOTS

Shot, shot, shot, shot. Not shots of liquor, but shots of drugs that crank Michelle's ovaries into overdrive, producing more and more follicles.

I play a small role in the process. Other than jerking off for sperm donations and keeping Michelle happy and upbeat about the process, it's giving her these shots. So I aim to get really good at it.

Today the dosage has changed. We give the shot every night at 6:00 p.m. And as usual, Puck moseys into the bathroom to watch. He likes most of the routine—everything except the pungent smell of the alcohol swab. I suspect it smells too much like his flea medicine. His nose bunches up and his whiskers fall back, unhappy with the stench.

I go into the bathroom and get "the pen." The pen is a plastic tube full of liquid drugs, in this case, Gonal F. On one end is a movable plastic dial and a plastic plunger that you can pull. On the other end is a rubber stopper like in bottles that you plunge needles in to get medicine. The needles for this step are small, a little larger than the ones used for insulin. It feels like I am doing DNA testing for a medical breakthrough. No, I'm just revving up my wife's baby maker.

Even though we may only have one day of shots left, we have no choice but to use a new pen. I prepare to prime it. I screw in the needle and turn the dosage meter to 37.5, which is the minimum. I won't be giving this dosage, but you have to prime the pen first to get the air out. I pull back the plunger and gently press it in until all the air escapes and a single drop of liquid slides down the end of the needle.

The first time I did this, the liquid shot to the ceiling. Puck saw it fly like a rocket and bolted from the room. He probably went to tell Michelle to run for it.

I am much less of an amateur now. I switch out the

needles, careful to sterilize the rubber tip. I turn the dosage meter to 150, tonight's dosage, and I call out to Michelle and tell her I am ready.

We've developed a routine for this. I am not going to say that I am an expert, but I've learned. I can tell Michelle doesn't dread these shots anymore.

She comes into the bathroom with an ice pack. I open the alcohol swab. Puck's nose twitches, his eyes squint and he darts from the room again.

Michelle holds the ice pack on her stomach for a few seconds and then I swab. I give these shots just below and to the side of her bellybutton. She either pinches a small bunch of flesh or stretches it out. She doesn't have a lot of flesh, so we've found that pinching hurts less. She pinches and I smoothly and quickly push the needle in. Not fast but with no hesitation.

I learned hesitation hurts when I tried it out on myself (with no medicine of course). I told Michelle I would give myself a shot every night if it would make her feel any better. She was nice enough to refuse my offer.

I make sure to hold the needle steady. A few times early on I would switch hands or turn my hand to dispense the drugs and when the needle shifts, a slice of pain accompanies it. I hold the needle with one hand and push the plunger in until I hear the last of the clicks, confirming that the proper dose has been completely dispensed inside Michelle. I gently, but again swiftly, extract the needle and cover the injection site with a cotton swab.

I feel guilty giving these shots. I know that I am

hurting her, even if it's just a little bit. While the pen is dispensing hormones, I am the one dispensing the pain.

LESSON 21: PRACTICE MAKES PERFECT.

INFERTILITY STORIES

You don't hear much about other people's fertility issues until you go through it yourself. Now it seems like every woman I talk to has a story—either her own, a family member's or a good friend's. I was on the phone with one of my clients this afternoon, and the subject of fertility treatments bubbled up. She had also been to the Texas Fertility Center and seen Dr. Vaughn. They went through five years of treatments (fortunately for them, they were at least covered by health insurance) before she and her husband decided to adopt. They never did figure out why she couldn't get pregnant.

The doubts creep in every additional month we don't get pregnant, and these stories don't help matters.

THE MILLER BASKETBALL TEAM

The gonadotropins must be furiously working on something in my body, because aside from feeling faint, especially in the sun, I'm constantly starving. I'm rarely hungry, so this is a new phenomenon to me. I eat every couple hours to no avail. Oh well. Now that I know that no amount of food is going to make my voracious appetite go away, I just need to steer clear of the pantry.

My stomach is protruding (please tell me that's just bloating!) and my pants are a little tight. And a few pimples have popped up on my face. I feel like an impressionable 14-year-old girl, riddled with acne, trying to eat away her problems. I doubt Chris will find this wildly attractive.

Our first check-up sonogram shows we have five follicles growing. My estradiol is a little higher than Dr. Vaughn would like at this point, so he suggests we cut the dose back from 150 IU to 75 IU per night.

The doc explains, "It's better to drive a fast car that you have to let up on the gas than a slow car that you can't get moving up the hill."

Dr. Vaughn tells us that my fast response to the injectables is a good sign. Apparently, injectables don't always work for women with higher FSH numbers.

Three days later, I'm feeling frisky from my surging estrogen level. I consider attacking Chris before work, but my need for more sleep takes precedence.

The next sonogram shows eight follicles, which are all growing steadily. My estradiol has tapered off to a level Dr. Vaughn's comfortable with.

My ovaries feel like they're full of lemons. We go in for what we expect to be our last sonogram a couple days later, but none of the now 13 follicles are big enough yet (the target size for a mature follicle is 20mm), so we'll have to come back again in two more days.

I don't think I've brought up the hassle of sonogram days. It's not just the time it takes to get through the doctor's appointments, but I also have to go in for a blood test before 8:00 a.m. on sonogram days to check my hormone levels. I don't have much room for complaint, since blood work days are usually the only days I actually have to set an alarm. I work for myself as a marketing consultant, and I never set up meetings before 10:00 a.m. if I have the choice. This is one of my favorite things about my job (that, along with the absence of corporate swindling, no pointless meetings, being able to go to work in my pajamas and Scooby Doo slippers, and working from the couch with the TV on).

***

Our final sonogram brings us a shock. All of my follicles grew a little more quickly over the last 48 hours than the doctor had expected. No wonder I felt like I'd been storing fruit in my ovaries. Chris and I were playing one-on-one soccer yesterday and I could feel the lemons bouncing around in there like the balls in a corn popper push toy.

I mention this to the nurse, when she informs me that I'm not supposed to do any heavy aerobic activities like running for precisely that reason.

Oops!

In stimulation cycles, the doctor's goal is to grow multiple follicles but to only have two or three at 20mm when the trigger shot is scheduled so that triplets are the biggest risk you'll face. Again, we are trying to avoid having The Brady Bunch.

But even with all the careful watching, the doctor warns us that we have five follicles big enough to fertilize, that we run a risk of multiples and asks if we want to proceed anyway. If we do find ourselves in the situation with too many fertilized embryos, we would need to undergo a reduction procedure at a special clinic in Houston. There they would pluck the lemons from my fertile tree.

I can't imagine having to deal with that, but Chris and I agree we'll cross that bridge if that's where the path takes us.

As an added bonus for our lousy timing, now we get to spend 20% extra for having our two IUIs over the weekend.

That night, Chris plunges the trigger shot—a vial of Ovidrel—into my stomach to induce ovulation. About 20 minutes later, I sprint to the bathroom with severe stomach cramps. About three hours later, my stomach finally relaxes and I'm able to go to sleep. The next morning, we're scheduled for the first IUI. We've been through the drill before, so we know what to expect this time with the plunger labeled "Miller."

***

The sonogram before our second IUI confirms that I've released two of my eggs and another follicle appears ready to release. The last two large follicles could release later today. This is why they schedule two IUIs—just in case the first one is too early. They want fresh sperm swimming around when the eggs enter the uterus.

The overweight 14-year-old in me is screaming for food, apparently from the change in my estrogen level. My legs are also aching enough to get in the way of my sleep, but maybe this is a test to make sure I am really ready for children. After all, I love sleep more than nearly any other activity in life. I can get nine to ten hours of sleep every night if something (my husband or our cats or an alarm or the neighbor's dog) doesn't wake me up beforehand.

There is one benefit to the amount of sleep I get each night—I'm never tired during the day. A Texas-sized lunch won't even put me out. And I might have a few less wrinkles around my eyes, since I typically get all the beauty rest I need (or is that just an old wives' tale?).

All we can do in the two weeks between our IUIs and our scheduled pregnancy test is wait. Chris and I argue about what we should and shouldn't say to our families. We agree not to worry them unnecessarily about the number of eggs that could fertilize.

I call my parents and tell them there were a few follicles that appeared to be the right size, only two of which had released. My mom says, "That's great news." Then there's silence. "Right?"

I laugh and tell her the only great news would be if I end up being pregnant after our first $3,500 in fertility treatments.

Chris' parents are even less in the loop, so we don't give them the play-by-play update. We figure we'll fill them in on the one thing they'll really care about—if and when we're finally pregnant!

Meanwhile, Chris and I joke about multiple births every chance we get. He'll write an email asking how our five children are. I'll write back asking him if he is getting in shape to be the 6th man on our Miller basketball team. On our walks, he'll start listing off all of the names he likes, just in case we have to be ready with more than one.

THERE IS NO I IN TEAM

My period arrives like clockwork on day 25, a few days before I was scheduled for a pregnancy test. What happened to our basketball team? I had high hopes that at least one of the eggs would fertilize.

One theory is that even if there were good embryos, they may not have had enough time to implant. Implantation can take anywhere from 8-12 days. Meanwhile, my luteal phase, the number of days between ovulation and the end of the cycle, is only 10 days. My doctor already knew I had short cycles. I reminded him anyway and I had mentioned it to the other doctor on call over the weekend when we had our IUIs and both dismissed the issue, explaining that the fertility medications usually take care of these things.

I bring it up again when I return for our next day 3 sonogram for round 2 of fertility treatments. After looking at the calendar and seeing that my period arrived early, the doctor says, "Hmmmm, well, we'll definitely put you on progesterone next time. I'll make a note in here, but you can remind me too."

The most dangerous weapon in my reach is a paperback book. I fire it at Dr. Vaughn and he dodges it with amazingly fast reflexes. Maybe he's secretly a superhero like Spiderman?

In reality, I just wring my hands and swear under my breath.

***

A week later, I'm watching an episode of *Gray's Anatomy*, happy that I'm not pregnant with five children. The entire show revolves around a woman who's just had quintuplets and four of the babies are fighting to survive through all kinds of structural issues, like underdeveloped lungs, a slow-beating heart and infections. The mother is torn apart knowing she had the choice to keep just two or three and dramatically increase the chances that they would all be born healthy. A lousy choice to have to make.

AN ODD DIVERSION

I'm at work one day when I go to the restroom and as the stream begins to flow, my penis burns furiously. It hurts so bad that I stop twice only realizing that it hurts more when it starts than just to continue.

I've never had any kind of issue at all with peeing, so I am worried. Also we have an injectables cycle coming up soon, and if this screws it up, we've just blown three grand.

I call Michelle and she sets up an appointment with a specialist for that same day. A few hours later, I'm anxiously waiting in a patient room, hoping the doctor can tell me what's going on.

I'm reading a fishing magazine when the doctor comes in. He asks me when it hurts and a few other questions. I tell him there is one other symptom. Sometimes when I pee, the muscle under my groin hurts.

"Wrong answer," he says.

I find this odd coming from a doctor. And suddenly I know I am in trouble.

"Have you ever had a prostate exam?" he asks.

"Nope," I reply. "But it hurts when I pee, not…"

"It could be transverse pain. You don't want to mess around with your prostate."

Time slows way down at this point and every ounce of my intellect searches for a way to stall the inevitable exam.

It is singularly the most uncomfortable thing I have ever experienced.

Fortunately, I didn't experience any dramatic pain. He told me later that they call it the "roof test" because if there's an issue, you'll jump to the roof out of pain.

I pull up my pants and try to salvage what part of my dignity I have left as he explains that it's likely an infection in my urethra. He'll prescribe both an antibiotic and a specific painkiller that will work nearly immediately.

"There is one side effect to it though." He explains, "It will turn your urine orange." Great—I'll be peeing Longhorn color. I don't care as long as it works and I don't have to bend over again.

LESSON 22: PROSTATE EXAMS SUCK.

TRIPLETS

I am at lunch with a friend today who asks me all about our fertility saga. She tells me about a friend of hers who is expecting triplets in a couple months. Triplets. Three crying children all at once. Three car seats. Three diapers full of poop. Three sets of clothes. Three bedrooms. Three cars at 16. Three college funds. My head swells up like a balloon, overwhelmed by threes. So even though I really want to get pregnant, please God let me only have one or at most two at one time! On my drive home, I zoom through three yellow lights still dizzy with the thought.

As a kid, I dreamed of having twins when I grew up. That was probably because at one point, I was infatuated with the lives of the two cool, blond identical twins in the *Sweet Valley High* series. But as I grew up and saw how much work kids were, that dream was shot to hell.

Twins do run in my family. And with the higher chances of having multiples with fertility drugs, I've accepted the fact that if I ever get pregnant, it could easily be with more than one. But only time will tell. First, I actually have to get pregnant.

We're in round 2 of injectables. It's a Friday at the end of August and we're waiting for the doctor in one of the patient rooms. Chris aims the warming light at me, demanding to know in his poor German accent, "Where are the plans? Where are the plans?" Then he proceeded to put on a three-act show with shadow puppets on the wall until Dr. Vaughn arrives.

We're hoping the follicles are close to the popping point because Chris is traveling on Wednesday. It would suck to have bunches of eggs ready and no sperm to join them.

The largest follicle is at 16mm (Damn—Chris won again. He picked 16 and I'd picked the over). The doc thinks we'll be ready for the ovulation shot on Sunday, which means a trip to St. David's hospital before 8:00 a.m. for the blood test (all the other labs are closed on Sundays) and an extra 20% for the sonogram. If the follicles are big enough, we'll do the IUI on Monday and Tuesday. Phew—we're cutting it awfully close.

That was the good news.

The bad news is that the doctor picks on my fibroid today, showing us why the half-inch sucker might be a problem.

I ask, "What do you think the likelihood is that the fibroid is what's causing me not to get pregnant?"

He answers, "It's hard to say. We like to presume a fibroid innocent until proven guilty, but if you were going to spend the money on IVF or more than three cycles of injectables, I would recommend having the surgery first."

This surgery, an abdominal myomectomy, requires a large incision, up to six weeks of recovery time and a C-section if we ever do have a baby to deliver.

As I'm writing this, I catch myself sighing out loud and realize that's exactly how I feel—full of sighs. Wouldn't it be nice if this process was a little easier? Every job I can think of seems like a cakewalk compared to this. I'm just ready to be pregnant.

Chris and I talk about the surgery on the way home and he can tell I'm a little depressed by the fibroid stuff. We decide it's best to try one more injectables cycle and one IVF cycle before resorting to surgery.

I call my mom and tell her the news. I desperately try to choke back the tears, but I'm drowning in a flood of emotions. My cries are soft and quiet so my mom won't hear. When she figures out that I'm not saying anything because I am sobbing, she starts crying too.

After we both settle down, she offers to pay for an

in vitro cycle if we need it. This makes me feel worlds better, because one of the worst-case scenarios in my mind is to spend more than $12,000 and end up with nothing to show for it other than a credit card bill.

If I'm a parent someday, I hope I can make my kids feel that they can always count on me in a crisis. That I'll always be there for them, no matter what. That's how my mom and dad make me feel.

***

It's Sunday. I find the hospital lab after making a few rounds on the wrong floor and then head home and straight back to bed.

A few hours later, the sonogram shows two follicles at more than 20mm (and one at 16mm, which apparently has about a 50% chance of releasing), so we're all set for the Ovidrel shot tonight and two IUI appointments tomorrow and Tuesday afternoon.

There's a message on our answering machine when we get home that my blood test shows a lower estrogen level and a higher progesterone count than expected, so the doctor believes I might ovulate today instead of tomorrow. They've changed our IUI appointment to Monday morning.

***

When the alarm goes off again at 7:00 a.m. for the IUI

collection and delivery, I groan and slump out of bed like a zombie.

I haven't spent much time on the whole sperm collection process. This is not a topic that most people want to hear about, so let me just say that the first couple of times we went through this, I wasn't much help. The cats jumping up and down off the bed didn't offer much assistance either. Nor did the time pressure.

Chris and I finally agree to a strategy going forward. I get him warmed up, he gets his sperm into the cup (don't miss!), and I drop it off.

I steal an hour nap between the sperm drop off and our doctor's appointment and then it's back to the clinic to see if the follicles have popped. Nope! The three follicles are still intact. Not what the doctor expected based on my blood test Sunday. But since he's expecting ovulation to occur soon, we proceed with the first IUI.

Chris watches as the doctor lets loose 40 million sperm into my uterus and we chat until the clock tells us it's been ten minutes and I'm free to get up.

***

One more IUI to go. I want to crush the alarm with a sledgehammer. We go through the same routine again and once the IUI process is complete, I savor the thought of seeing no doctors for two whole weeks.

Dr. Vaughn has prescribed progesterone for this

round. That regiment will start Friday and continue until two weeks from today, when I'll head over for a blood test to see if I'm pregnant. There's only one small problem. I haven't received the progesterone yet.

FedEx never showed up and the online pharmacy claims that someone named P. Howell signed for it. I check to make sure they have the right date and the right address and then declare that it must have been delivered to the wrong place because I am the only Howell at this address and I never received it. After an arduous run-around, the clinic transfers my prescription to a local pharmacy and I pick up the progesterone in time to take it that morning.

The FedEx guy arrives an hour later and explains that he did, in fact, deliver it to the wrong address. The guy who signed for it just assumed it was his roommate's package. He apologizes and smiles, saying, "They did refrigerate it though."

Great—still fresh. Too bad I don't need it anymore.

My belly is bloated and I'm constipated. Every step I take hurts my stomach. But after lots of fiber and a couple long walks, I'm almost back to normal. All of these trials and tribulations better be worth it.

SCHOOL SPIRIT

I'm at a Texas Football game and it's a close, exciting game. I've had too much to drink, of water that is, so I run to the restroom during the TV time out.

There's a very long line of slightly inebriated fans waiting. Insults and Texas Fight echo through the bathroom.

Finally a urinal opens up and I step up to do my business. As I let loose my stream, I have a private chuckle about the fact that my pee is burnt orange.

I finish and step to the sink to wash my hands and I hear the drunken fan using the urinal I just left shouting.

"Now THAT is school spirit, that dude pees orange!"

A bunch of people look at him like he's nuts.

I run back to my seat thinking about how many invisible lines we have crossed. How many odd things now seem perfectly routine? Other than destroying my dignity and a compliment from a fan, I'm just not sure we've really gotten anywhere. I go back and forth day-by-day.

Sometimes I think it is inevitable, that we must be close, and sometimes I think we're no closer and all we have done is compromised tiny pieces of ourselves.

LESSON 23: I AM A SUPER FAN. I CAN PEE BURNT ORANGE.

STRIKE TWO

It is the 5ᵗʰ Anniversary of 9/11, which would be depressing enough without the added fact that I'm spotting this morning. The doctor had said most women will not begin bleeding until after they stop the progesterone, so I'm not sure if this indicates a problem.

I did hear a "happy" infertility story this morning. A friend of my sister's called to offer her support. Her story was similar to several others I'd heard. She was 30 years old when she started trying and she had a slightly elevated FSH (12—the same as mine). She tried Clomid, went through three cycles of injectables with IUIs, and forked out the money for two in vitro cycles before getting pregnant. When they went back to the doctor to try for a second pregnancy, her doctor said there was less than a 5% chance of success, as her ovaries showed clear signs of "slowing down" (that's the euphemism for crapping out). She went off to acupuncture, took some herbs she read about online, and got pregnant on her own—two more times. She is the mother of three healthy children.

Nice to hear a story like that, especially on a day like today, because as of this afternoon, I know I'm not pregnant (the cramps are back to torture my soul and my stomach). It's a disappointing, all too familiar feeling.

I guess I can cross the pregnancy test off my list of things to do tomorrow. All I can do is move forward, so I call the doctor's office to schedule a day 2 or day 3 sonogram for the next round.

ONE MORE TRY

Chris can't make it to my sonogram appointment, so I'm waiting in the lobby alone reading a book. I look around the waiting room of the new clinic, with marble floors and leather chairs throughout. I think they're making enough money. They could have furnished the whole room with my payments alone.

In the exam room, I'm literally shaking from the air conditioning cascading out of the vents above. Apparently they are still working on regulating the temperature throughout the office. They're certainly making enough money to hire an AC guy to check things out?

No cysts this time, so we'll give the injectables one more try, especially since our online pharmacy offers the drugs free on your third try.

Yeah—a financial break!

I check with the doctor to make sure starting my period while still on progesterone doesn't indicate a larger problem, but he says it did its job—lengthening my luteal phase to 13 days instead of 10.

The same FedEx guy arrives with my medication box later that day and exclaims, "I got the right house this time!" I laugh and sign for the package. If I keep this fertility stuff up, I'll have to put the delivery guys on our Christmas list.

The third injectables cycle is similar to the last two and all the shots, drug side effects, blood tests, sonograms, heavy ovaries are old hat. Two of the follicles are big enough to take the Ovidrel shot and our first IUI goes off without a hitch. I ask the doctor to check to see if the fibroid has grown since I've started on fertility medication. Nope—still 15mm.

***

The next morning, my alarm is set for 7:10 a.m. I wake up to a room that seems lighter than it should be and lo and behold, my alarm clock flashes 12:00 a.m. but the cable box shows it is 7:34 a.m. Crap! Nothing like a little time pressure. Chris jokes that we can fool around in the car on the way to the doctor's office. We don't try that. I make it to the office only six minutes late.

A few hours later, the sonogram indicates that three follicles have released. One of the follicles looks large and different than the rest. The doctor explains that it has blood inside, which he assures us is common. That's probably why my right side has been hurting.

***

My period is later than usual and I feel a little nauseous. Could this finally be it? Third time's a charm, right?

Wrong. More like three strikes and you're out.

My period comes. Our hopeful injectables cycle #3 ends the same way as #1 and #2. No baby. Just cramps, cramps and more cramps.

I feel deflated and pissed and frustrated and ready to throw something. But none of those things will change the fact that I'm not pregnant.

ADVICE

Michelle has started to get extremely frustrated with the advice our family and friends are giving. Even strangers offer nuggets. Yes, people really do advise us to get drunk or go on vacation and eat ice cream.

I see it as a sign that they care. Michelle, on the other hand, is not appreciative of any of the suggestions offered. To her, it's just someone talking nonsense that doesn't know what it feels like to be in her shoes. It doesn't matter that they're trying to be supportive—she still wants to shut it out.

We're with our friends who are also heading down the fertility treatment path. Michelle's listening to a story about a girl complaining it took her two months to get pregnant that begins with "bitch" and ends with "the girl should try to drink a little less." It's then that I realize Michelle is actually taking infertility stuff very well. I've since heard stories about other women dealing with infertility by breaking all the china, sobbing on the floor, and screaming incessantly at anyone and everyone. So I am reminded that it can always be worse.

LESSON 24: IF SOMEONE GIVES YOU ADVICE, REMEMBER THEY ARE ACTUALLY TRYING TO HELP.

DECISION TIME

It's decision time. The question is if I should try one IVF cycle first or have an abdominal myomectomy to remove the fibroid. My doctor's recommending the latter. I'd been leaning toward the former until a couple days ago, when I read an article about in vitro success with and without fibroid complications (the success logically being greater without the complications). Not to mention the issues of fibroids causing miscarriages.

It's also going to be nearly impossible to squeeze in one IVF try and, if it doesn't work, then the myomectomy surgery before year-end. And even if we could squeeze it in, this would mean cancelling our Thanksgiving, Christmas and New Year's vacations already planned. Before year-end is important, because I'd like to take advantage of the fact that there's only $700 left before I reach my out of pocket maximum on our health insurance plan this year. I'd much rather pay $700 for the surgery than $3,500.

So we're forgoing an IVF try first and I'm now on the doctor's surgery schedule for October 24th.

My mother has sent me at least 30 articles on fibroids in the last week and is begging me to get a second opinion. This is classic Dr. Howell stuff and she isn't letting it go, no matter how much I ignore her. It would be nice to have someone else tell me a myomectomy is exactly what we should do next, but where I'm going to get a solid second opinion in the next two weeks is beyond me, especially since we're heading out on vacation for a week this coming Friday. I'm buried under a heaping pile of decisions, along with work and personal to-do lists. After yet another call from my mom, who appears to have gotten my sister involved, I concede to a second opinion. At least it will stop the barrage of hounding and emails.

A SECOND OPINION

We decide to get a second opinion. Well, we don't really decide—Michelle's mom and sister colluded and made an appointment for us to see a fertility specialist in San Antonio and we acquiesced.

We arrive in the office. It is teeming with people, nearly every chair taken. Compared to our "fertility hotel," this place feels like a clinic. No fish tank. No high end comfy couches. Just hard plastic chairs, pale colored walls, overrun magazine racks and linoleum tile.

When we check in at the large wooden desk, I notice a woman anxiously hovering. We find two seats across the room and I start to wonder what she is waiting for. And then the door flies open. In charges a heavy-set man, drenched in sweat. The woman's face lights up. She's flailing her hands, encouraging her husband to run. The big lug slumps to the front desk. I thought he was going to collapse in the middle of the hallway.

I am about to let out a rattling scoff to assert my disapproval at this woman making a scene, when her cherry-faced, sweating husband, plops a paper bag on the desk. A thick wave of relief flushes across his face. Mission accomplished. The woman at the desk whisks the paper bag, and the wife, through a door.

My scoff morphs into a laugh-snort. And I realize when everyone looks at me that it was out loud. Gosh, I'm such an ass. I want to tell everyone, 'Hey, been there, done that.' But, instead I bury my head in a magazine.

A half hour later we are in the doctor's office giving our synopsis of our fertility saga. He hadn't received Michelle's file but it is being faxed over as we speak.

He knows Dr. Vaughn. In fact, he was Dr. Vaughn's protégé. He tells us he would trust Dr. Vaughn and that it is likely that he is right, but if we really want his opinion he can do a test called a <u>hysterosalpingo contrast sonography</u>. Something about a balloon and some dye. Sounds like a blast. Sure, what the heck.

Michelle lies down on the table and I get to watch her go through yet another painful, or at least extremely uncomfortable looking experience.

The doctor ultimately ends up with a picture of the fibroid, which is completely embedded in the wall. He assures us that the myomectomy surgery is the only option to remove it.

We ask him if this could impact pregnancy and he says yes. But more importantly, he says if Michelle gets pregnant, it may cause complications that could lead to a miscarriage.

We decide that we don't need to experience one of those.

LESSON 25: DR. VAUGHN WAS RIGHT. AGAIN.

MORE QUESTIONS, BUT NO NEW ANSWERS

I keep thinking this fibroid is so small, but when you see it on an ultrasound screen, it looks like the iceberg that shipwrecked the Titanic. Our "second opinion doctor" is silent throughout the test (maybe because there really is an iceberg in my vagina). Then he confirms that the majority—85-90%—of the fibroid, is in fact inside the lining and not inside the cavity.

We go back into his office and he confirms Dr. Vaughn's recommendation. The fibroid should be removed.

Would it be reasonable to try an IVF cycle if we had all the money in the world? Sure.

Would it be reasonable to go ahead and get the fibroid out before trying IVF? You betcha.

Then I mention what's been bothering me the most. Pointing to his doodle of my fibroid, I explain that I don't believe this can be the primary reason for my infertility because there's an awful large area where an embryo could have implanted at this point.

So I ask.

Me: "Can the fibroid be impacting anything besides implantation in the area where it's nudging up against the cavity?"

Doctor: "Sure."

Me: "Like what?"

Doctor: "We don't really know. It could be preventing the egg from meeting the sperm. It could impact sperm motility. It could be messing with your hormones. We just don't know."

I sigh under my breath and wonder if we'll ever have a definitive answer on why it's been two years and several fertility treatments later and we still aren't pregnant.

I'll be going under the knife in a week.

REMINDERS EVERYWHERE

There's an extremely pregnant woman at the pool in a bikini today. She is so big, if she did a jump off the diving board the baby would probably fall out. We are a little unnerved. She is fit and attractive, but the bikini is desperately trying to stretch out and cover the full surface area and it's failing miserably. She might as well be completely naked. (Well, okay, that might be slightly more unnerving—especially around all of the children, and their fathers.)

I can't stand it anymore. I sprint over and throw a towel around her while screaming out, "PLEASE, OH PLEASE, COVER THAT BELLY!" She looks at me like I've gone crazy, yanks off the towel and runs to the pool. She yells out, "FREEDOM!" before she jumps into the water cannonball-style.

The splash of a child jumping into the pool breaks me out of my daydream and I see the scarcely clad pregnant lady still stretched out in the sun.

Until I wanted a child, I never noticed how many pregnant women there are. They're everywhere I look. In the grocery store. In the park. Walking down the street. Working out at the gym. Women with little round bellies just on that border, where you're not sure if you should say congratulations and so you keep your mouth shut and just smile. Women who are clearly pregnant, but appear to still be adjusting to the bowling ball shape in their midsection. And by adjusting, I mean ditching the bikini for a full-bodied swimsuit. Then there are those with oversized watermelon bellies, like the woman at the pool. How do they tie their shoes with a little person in the way now? I hope to know someday.

It's not just the pregnant women either. The same can be said for babies and children. They're everywhere I look. They even run around in my dreams now.

UNDER THE KNIFE

I'm going through the details on the abdominal myomectomy with the nurse. She doesn't dive very deep regarding the actual surgery—just covers the basics about what I should expect in terms of recovery.

She explains that if all goes well, I should expect to be in the hospital for three to five days and then rest at home for an additional three to four weeks. Four weeks for recovery seems crazy. I ask her if it will really be a month, or if that's just a worst-case scenario.

"Some people recover faster, but in general, Dr. Vaughn recommends taking four weeks off from work and if you're feeling better after three weeks, then you can go back early." Her stock answer leaves me feeling pessimistic.

I read through several forums on the surgery to gather more feedback. All I uncover are disastrous stories where people were still struggling to recover after three months or six months or even years. They're listless and tired. They don't have enough energy to exercise. They can't sleep. They're constantly in pain.

What am I getting myself into? My stomach feels like it's filled with volcano lava. A tiny part of me considers packing our bags and traveling around Europe for a year.

Chris and I have several "if I die" discussions. I even write him a goodbye note that's hidden in my sock drawer in case something goes very wrong (like the doctor leaving a scalpel in my ovaries, which they don't find until my autopsy).

One of Chris' favorite topics is whom he's allowed to sleep with if I'm gone. Really? This could be one of our last conversations and Chris chooses the topic of sex. What a surprise. He detests my "no sleeping with married women" rule, but at least he's agreed to staying away from girls under 21.

Laura is coming in for the day to see me a few hours after the surgery is over. My mother meanwhile keeps telling me she's cleared her calendar and is expecting to come the day after my surgery to take over. When we'd talked about it last, I said, "If I'm not feeling great by the end of the week, I'd love for you to come." Somehow that turned into her coming no matter the case.

Oh well—if I'm feeling terrible, that will be great. And if I'm feeling great, she won't have to get on a plane.

It's a week until Halloween and my surgery is less than 12 hours from now. (Note: All the fun of Halloween gets sucked out when you are actually being cut open like one of Freddy Krueger's big-boobed victims.) I really should stop watching TV and pack for the hospital, but it seems so much easier to continue lounging on the couch. Chris just paused the DVR on the Dallas Cowboy cheerleaders. Now he's rewinding in slow motion to watch their chests jiggle up and down like Jell-O bowls the size of melons. While he is a boob guy, he's mostly doing this to pick at my resolve. I don't take the bait. This is my cue to get my act together and head to bed, especially since we have to be at the hospital by 5:30 a.m.

***

When the alarm goes off, it feels like I only just drifted off to sleep. It is pitch black outside. Nobody's supposed to be up at this time in the morning, except maybe the owl that's hooting as we drag ourselves into the car and head to the hospital to check in. I smile at the sound—maybe it's a sign of good luck.

When we arrive, I peer at the other families in the

waiting room and thank God that I'm here for something voluntary and fixable. They call my name and I put on my old friend the hospital gown. How many of these will I have to wear in my lifetime?

The nurse comes in to put a nametag on my arm and get the IV started and Chris continues to entertain me while we wait.

I'm nervous and my empty stomach lurches. I'm not worried about never waking up from the anesthesia since I've been "under" before. But you just never know with surgeries—even the routine ones. It sure would suck to die from an elective procedure. I'd imagine the only thing worse would be dying from liposuction or breast implants.

I try to picture how Chris would deal with my untimely demise. I have to say, I think he'd be pretty crushed, which would make me sadder than the unhappiness I'd feel no longer being among the living. I don't have much more time to contemplate, as the anesthesiologist arrives to add a sleepy concoction to my IV. The last thing I remember is kissing Chris goodbye.

SECOND SURGERY

It's hard to believe she's doing this again. It's never easy watching someone you love get wheeled into surgery. No matter how clinical the hospital is, there is a strong emotional connection that dissects through all the sterile lights and procedures.

I again say goodbye to my wife, wondering if at some point this will actually be worth it.

I realize that in all of my humor, in all of my keeping Michelle positive, I'm beginning to doubt. Not just if we'll ever be able to have a kid. But wondering if it's worth the risk. I'm happy to live my life with at least Michelle, but not ever without her.

They turn the corner and Michelle's gurney disappears into the labyrinth.

I steel myself against my thoughts. I have to stay positive. I, actually we, have committed to this course.

LESSON 26: THE DOUBTS ARE BOUND TO CREEP IN AT SOME POINT.

GROANING IS BAD

I wake up to a very bright light.

Waking up is good.

I can hear myself groaning in pain.

Groaning is bad.

I'm having trouble breathing, I'm bombarded with constant waives of nausea and I can feel tears streaming down the sides of my face. The nurse asks me if I'm in pain. I scream. Then the blackness takes over again.

The next time I wake is more pleasant. Whatever drug the nurse gave me seems to have taken effect and by the time they're ready to roll me to my room, I'm in great spirits.

That euphoria doesn't last very long.

When I move from the surgery bed to the stationary bed in my recovery room, it feels like my stomach has been ripped open with a can opener.

But once I settle in again and don't move, there is only a little pain. The oxygen tube over my face is a little annoying and the catheter is downright icky, but I'm alive and fibroid-free, and Chris is by my side to cheer me up. I don't have much to complain about.

When my sister arrives, she sits down next to my

bed, takes my hand and starts to cry. I must look like a disaster. I'm sure the oxygen tube streaming from my nose doesn't help.

I should be taking pictures to document the great lengths I'm going through to have a child. There will be no, "When I was young, we used to have to walk two miles in the snow to get to school" lecture. I'll have even better guilt material. "See, this is from when Mommy had her uterus opened up by a pair of pliers. This one is when Mommy had a Macy's Day Parade balloon inflated in her vagina." And I'm sure there will be great material from future sacrifices before he or she is even born.

Laura stays for a few hours and we chat while Chris escapes the hospital to grab us lunch. She'll come back to take care of me for a day or two when I get home from the hospital and Chris has returned to work.

GOODBYE FIBROID

Michelle is out of surgery. She has a tube in her nose, she's doped up on drugs and I can tell that she will be in pain when they wear off. Her stomach is so swollen and bloated, she could be pregnant. But of course I know better. She slips in and out of sleep.

But at least she no longer has a fibroid to worry about. I wonder what they do with it? I should have asked them to save it in a jar for us. Someday I could say, "This is the fibroid Mommy had taken out of her uterus so she could have you!" Then they'd look back at me like I was crazy. And they'd be right to an extent. Aren't we all a little crazy?

Her sister has called twice and she'll walk through the door at any moment.

Michelle opens her eyes and asks me to bring her some water. There have been way too many jokes at my expense about me not being able to take care of Michelle, so I reply, "Oh my gosh, milk it why don't you. How long are you going to keep this up?"

Michelle's mouth opens to respond, but then she sees me smile.

I go to get her a glass of water and an icepack for her head. Her sister peeks in the door.

Laura whispers delicately, "Hi. How is she doing?"

I think she presumes Michelle is sleeping.

"She's doing well." I reply in a normal voice.

Laura enters the room, taking the full scene in, and begins to sob. I think it is the tube in Michelle's nose, which makes her look worse than she is.

Seeing how much she cares about Michelle brings tears to my eyes. She hugs Michelle and somehow it is Michelle making Laura feel better, not the other way around. This is bizarre, but it's exactly the way families work.

I leave to get lunch for all of us. I hope that Laura can keep Michelle's mind off of "trying" for at least a few hours. I want her to focus on getting better first. The next step after a full recovery will be the most powerful fertility option of all—in vitro.

LESSON 27: KEEP COLLECTING THOSE STORIES TO TELL YOUR KIDS SOME DAY.

ON THE MEND

Dr. Vaughn arrives in my hospital room later that evening and explains that the surgery went just as expected. He says even if the fibroid wasn't impacting fertility, it might have caused problems after getting pregnant. With the increased hormone levels during pregnancy, fibroids can grow much bigger. The good news is that he never had to go inside the uterine cavity, so scar tissue shouldn't be an issue.

Since I'm feeling pretty good and Dr. Vaughn knows I want to go home as soon as possible, he stops the automatic pain medicine through the IV drip. I'll have to push the magic button if I need it. (I wish life could be this way—when it gets too overwhelming, just push a button.) But my pain remains steady at about a 3 or 4 out of 10 (the catheter being the most painful), so I never get desperate enough to push it.

Luckily, I'm not at all hungry because my hospital dinner is water and an orange slushy.

Chris has been given no choice but to stay with me in the hospital room. There's something about not being able to get out of bed that makes me too nervous to be on my own. I can hear him snoring on the couch while I try to escape into the blackness of sleep. With the nurses coming in every few hours to take my blood and check my oxygen levels, and a machine beeping in warning that my IV has run out—twice—I wouldn't say I had much in the way of quality sleep. But I probably got the equivalent of a few power naps.

My latest nap comes to a grinding halt when I'm woken up to have the catheter removed at 6:45 a.m. What a glorious feeling that was (not the actual removal itself, but the relief of that damn thing being out of me).

Every time Chris hears a nurse come in, he asks if he can sleep a little longer. At 8:30 a.m. the nurse tries to talk me into taking a Vicodin. But I know that makes me nauseous, and my stomach isn't an issue at this point, so I'm extremely reluctant. I ask her to check with Dr. Vaughn to see if (a) I have to take pain medication at all and (b) if the answer is yes, if I can take a Tylenol 3 instead, since I know that has minimal side effects for me.

Before the nurse has an answer, Dr. Vaughn comes in to check on me and agrees that I certainly shouldn't take any pain medicine if I don't feel like I need it. I'll recover faster without them.

He peeks under the hood and confirms that everything looks good so far. I've got permission to eat whatever I want in small, bird-like quantities. And once I've hobbled up and down the hospital hallway a couple times, I'll have permission to go home. He's already signed for my release. I'm thrilled with the news that I could be going home after only one hospital night given the expectation they'd initially set at four or five nights.

Getting out of bed is a little uncomfortable; walking is more than a little uncomfortable. It feels like a knife is slicing through my gut and my insides are all shoving up against each other like shoppers standing outside Walmart on Black Friday. But all in all, I was expecting much worse.

I'm home on the couch by 10:00 a.m., 24 hours after my surgery was completed.

I take some walks from the front of the house to the back of the house with my shoulders hunched over, but otherwise, the couch is my best friend.

When I'm allowed to take my first shower, the hot water feels fantastic. I think back and laugh that, as a kid, I hated taking showers. I can't recall why that was now, but I remember turning the shower on, wasting a bunch of water while sitting on a chair (outside the shower) and waiting an appropriate amount of time to be believable that I'd actually gotten clean. My mom finally caught me once and that was the end of the fake showers. Maybe I was a cat in a former life? Today, the shower feels like a giant slice of heaven.

With relaxation as our goal, Laura and I accomplish a lot over the next two days. We watch six episodes of *Studio 60*, write our Christmas lists, eat Kitchen Door chicken salad sandwiches, make some gold bars (delicious bars of yumminess made of eggs, yellow cake mix, cream cheese, confectioners sugar and butter— very low in fat as you can tell by the ingredients) and catch up on life.

I am feeling so good that I call the doctor's office to see if I can go for a walk outside. Their reply—"That's a bad idea." The nurse warns me that if I overdo it, I'll feel terrible and that will put me two steps back. Oh well, back to my rounds from the front of the house to the back of the house.

Every day I'm feeling better and better. The only pain left is when I cough or sneeze. I'm walking upright now, instead of hunched over. It doesn't even feel weird to get up off the couch anymore (moving my legs over the side first is no longer a required maneuver).

***

It's Saturday and Chris picks up Pappasita's fajitas for lunch—one of my all-time favorites. We watch football all day and tense up as UT gets behind 21-0 to Texas Tech up in Lubbock. Luckily, the horns pull out the win.

I take my first stroll on Saturday night, a week after the surgery. It feels refreshing out in the cold air. Then it feels even better to snuggle up in bed and sleep on my stomach.

***

On Sunday, we get up and go for a brisk walk, then head to the grocery store to stock up the fridge. That's when I start to feel a tugging inside my body, almost like a stitch in my side, but not in my side. It gets worse and worse the longer I stand. Not pain really, but definitely an uncomfortable feeling, like the way you feel after a big Thanksgiving meal.

So I tuck my tail in between my legs like a sad puppy and take it easy the rest of the day, watching Vince Young and the Titans beat up on the Texans. I also get some much-needed Christmas shopping done online. I'll take it easy tomorrow and then I'll be ready to get out and about on Tuesday night for the Texas Basketball season opener, which I'd been hoping to be well enough to attend before the surgery and now looks like a sure thing.

Then we can try again.

PART III

BRINGING IN THE BIG GUNS
(VIA THE SMALL PETRI DISH)

A NEW YEAR

It's a new year and someone in the family is pregnant, but it isn't me. My sister calls and drops the big news in my lap. She's due in July. I'm truly ecstatic for them, and if I get pregnant through IVF, then our kids will be about the same age.

It's time to begin our first IVF cycle, which starts with 21 days of birth control pills. What kind of backwards way of getting pregnant is that? The short explanation is that the fertility doctors want your ovaries completely shut down before over-stimulating them with drugs.

We're in Maui on vacation and I can't remember the

directions on when to start the pills. The time difference makes it impossible to reach anyone at the doctor's office back in Austin. So, I start the pills on day 1. Upon our return to Austin, we discover that I wasn't supposed to start taking them until day 3 or day 5. Crap. I've already managed to mess up our IVF cycle and we haven't even started the drugs yet. The nurse assures me it isn't a big deal.

**

I've made a long list of questions for our first IVF appointment with the doctor. The most important ones are around the experience of the IVF lab personnel and embryologist since their new lab will only have been open a few days before my egg retrieval.

Dr. Vaughn allays my fears. They are just moving the same lab personnel to their new location. Phew—we won't be the guinea pigs. Now we only have to worry that the lab is set up properly in terms of equipment, temperature, etc.

After our appointment, we get a lesson on <u>Lupron</u> shots. Luckily, these are very similar to my very dear friends the Gonal F shots, so we aren't too concerned about the administration. Lupron is used in IVF cycles to shut down the ovaries, giving total control to your doctor and the other drugs to manage ovulation. A Google search uncovers several nasty, possibly long-term side effects including memory loss, severe headaches and symptoms of stroke. Just what I needed—something new to worry about.

Once the shot lessons are over and we have our instructions, the "finance" person (i.e. she who takes our money) arrives to go over the laundry list of bills and when we'd need to pay them. She is whispery and apologetic at the start of the conversation, but when I let her know the figures weren't stressing us too much because my parents were paying for this round (thank you, thank you, thank you Mom and Dad!), she perks right up.

***

The next day is my first Lupron shot and for some reason Chris decides to "try it fast" this morning. It feels like I am being murdered with a syringe.

He says, "Hmmm—I was trying something new. I guess that doesn't work as well."

No. Definitely not.

I'll take Lupron for five days and then get another sonogram to make sure all is well (i.e. there are no cysts). If we get the okay, then we'll start on the Gonal F shots to crank up manufacturing on my eggs while continuing the Lupron shots for five more days.

Oh goodie—two shots a day!

IN VITRO IT IS

The cost of each IVF cycle will be about $12,000 for the drugs and procedures. The process is extensive, but at least there are some similarities to the injectables cycles we've already been through. And the benefit is that we should learn more and hopefully get pregnant in the process.

Everything seems different; there is a lot more pressure now. The schedule is much more rigorous. The shots are supposed to be given within 15 minutes of each other every night. The appointments are just as frequent until the eggs have grown. And then there are two BIG appointments—one for retrieval and one for implantation.

There is much less waiting and much more rushing—even at the doctor's office. I feel like I'm running a marathon to get my wife pregnant. I learn from being late to the first appointment not to be late for the next one. Michelle is already in the room and I have to shuffle back alone. It's very different alone, and not just because no one asks if I need to use the restroom. I feel like everyone is watching me. The last time that happened, I was in San Antonio and being glared at for laughing at the poor schmuck sprinting to deliver his sperm.

The in vitro process in simplified terms is as follows. Chemicals make sure that Michelle's body produces plenty of follicles, which when big enough, release eggs. This time, we want her to have as many eggs as possible—the more the better. We then give her a trigger shot full of a hormone that releases the eggs. Exactly 36 hours later, we'll go in for retrieval. The doctor will collect the eggs and then I will go into my little room. They'll combine her eggs and my sperm in petri dishes and then either three or five days later, they'll insert the best quality embryos back into Michelle's uterus. It's basically the same procedure performed in Jurassic Park, except we're hoping for a human baby instead of a T-Rex.

That is assuming that there are embryos. With as long as we have been trying without success, I might settle for a baby pterodactyl. Clearly, I am getting desperate.

LESSON 28: THE PRESSURE GROWS WITH TIME.

ANOTHER SPECIALIST

I've been going to acupuncture on and off over the last year. Since it hasn't worked yet, and with the IVF cycle coming up, I decide to find an acupuncture clinic that focuses mainly on reproductive issues.

I walk away from my first visit at the Cornerstone Acupuncture Center feeling like I have an IQ in the 20s. And I usually feel pretty smart compared to your average bear.

Instead of going straight into acupuncture, this clinic requires a consultation appointment first. And by consultation appointment, I mean an interrogation and a third grade biology lesson all in one. After the owner, David, introduced me to the concept of Qi (pronounced "Chi"), the conversation went something like this:

David: "What's an example of one of the systems in our body?"

Me: (after a few minutes, thinking it was a trick) "Uh, lymphatic?"

David: "Okay—that one's a little obscure. What about some others?"

Me: "Hmmm…"

David: "What moves all the blood around in our bodies?"

Me: "Uh…"

David: "The circulatory system. And what system is responsible for converting the food we eat into energy?"

Me: (without any confidence at this point) "The digestive system?"

David: "Right. And while there are a lot of parts involved in each system, there's one primary organ responsible. For example, what's the primary organ involved in the respiratory system?"

Me: (I can't recall what I answered here, but I mumbled something lame like the esophagus or bronchials.)

David: "It's the lungs. Did you skip biology class a lot when you were younger? (Lungs seems obvious to me now, but at the time I couldn't have answered correctly if he had one of his acupuncture needles aimed at my eye.)

Me: (meekly) "No. Actually, I was planning to go to medical school…"

David: (staring at me like I was the dumbest person alive) "Okay, let's move on."

David talked about how acupuncturists often look at the tongue for answers to what might be going on in the body. (I'm pretty sure all he will be able to tell is that I ate a blue raspberry Popsicle after lunch.) The shape of my tongue is apparently okay, but the coloring is a little white and uneven. It looks pretty standard pinkish to me (except when it's Popsicle blue). He says he can help, but that I'm a complex case. Hmmm. I wonder if "complex case" means expensive.

I don't have a known problem, so they'll have to keep tweaking the treatment to see what works. David recommends coming three times a week and twice on the day of the embryo transfer. Research studies have shown that receiving acupuncture treatments before and after the embryo transfer almost double IVF success rates. This was one of the main reasons I sought out experts in the field of acupuncture.

David seems to know what he's talking about and he certainly knows more biology than I can recall (although at this point, it's likely that a third grader knows more than I do, so he doesn't get too many bonus points for that). One month of treatment is $1,000 with a pay-up-front 20% discount, but in the scheme of things, IVF being more than $12,000, that doesn't seem like a high price to pay to increase my odds.

CHINESE MEDICINE

Since we still have no idea what has caused our fertility issues, Michelle has been spending more time online researching. Some of this research revolves around acupuncture and most of the articles show significantly improved IVF results, and fertility results in general, with this alternative medicine therapy.

I've always been curious about acupuncture, but it seems a little hokey that needles could solve so many problems.

There is an acupuncture clinic that specializes in fertility and Michelle already has an appointment. I make fun of her, but she doesn't care. She's willing to try almost anything at this point.

When she returns from her first appointment, she says, "I talked to the acupuncturist about you."

"What? Why did you talk about me? There is nothing wrong with me."

"I told him you were a skeptic. And that you thought this was a waste of time."

I do feel that way, but I didn't think I'd been so obvious. "What did he say?"

"That lots of people are skeptical but that if it didn't work, it wouldn't still be around 3,000 years later." I'm sure that's what psychics say, too.

And then Michelle explained that in acupuncture, the belief is that energy flows through your body and that sometimes this energy gets interrupted. Each system in our bodies has its own energy channel, called a meridian, which flows through the body. Different systems counterbalance each other. And each system can be too hot or too cold, too damp or too dry. The meridian, or pathway for each system, has different points along it to control the heat, cold, wet, and dry aspects. Placing needles at different points along the body helps restore these meridians, thereby restoring energy flow to all of our systems.

The whole concept of systems and meridians makes sense. But there are still lots of questions.

"So how the hell do they figure out what's wrong with you?" I quip.

Michelle has to ponder this for a second. I think I stumped her on this one. "He looked at my tongue and took my pulse."

Seriously? I could have done that for you at zero cost. "And what did he say was wrong with you?"

"My heart system is cold."

Michelle is always cold, but this could have been a lucky guess. Maybe her fingernails were blue. Or she was wearing a sweater in a Texas summer. There are plenty of telltale signs that probably tipped him off.

***

It's allergy season in Austin and my head feels like it's being squished under a steamroller. Michelle has been going to acupuncture three times a week and one day she comes home with a surprise. She told the acupuncturist that I had allergies and he gave her a tincture—a concoction of herbs brewed together like tea—for me to try.

David explained to her that the digestive system is

typically at the root of allergies. Makes sense actually. Whenever I have allergies, my stomach begins to ache.

I'm still a skeptic at this point, but his explanation captures my attention. I try the tincture. A few droppers full under my tongue and then I gulp it down, trying not to smell it. It tastes like muddy water filtered through an old boot.

Amazingly, over the next couple of days my symptoms dissipate. Now I'm curious enough to make an appointment.

This just makes me realize how little we know about everything, including why we can't get pregnant.

LESSON 29: THIS CRAZY ACUPUNCTURE STUFF REALLY WORKS.

IVF #1 IN FULL SWING

It's the day before Valentine's Day and we're heading to yet another sonogram. How romantic. Chris is acting his age—which for today is about 13. He begins by trying to start a punching match in the elevator. (God help us if we have a sensitive girl). Then he uses the heat lamp as a pretend microphone as if he's Mick Jagger belting out rock tunes. Have I mentioned that Chris doesn't have the best singing voice? And just before the doctor arrives, it's time for a spin on the doctor's stool. Chris feels so nauseous that he can barely stand. Serves him right, the little turd.

The doctor arrives and eyes Chris with a curious glance, unsure of my very peculiar husband. We stifle our laughter. We got what we came here for—the green light to start the follicle stimulation shots and get the IVF process moving.

***

Our next sonogram a couple days later shows slow growth of the follicles. In our past three injectables cycles, we'd had about ten follicles and at the first sonogram, which ranged from 4-8mm in size. So we were surprised to see fewer follicles, and smaller follicles, than our previous averages.

Dr. Vaughn explains that the Lupron, which I will still be on for a few more days, counteracts the Gonal F and therefore the slower growth is something he fully expects to see.

***

The next sonogram shows more follicles—eight this time—and steady growth and we're halfway home. At this sonogram appointment, Dr. Vaughn also does a mock transfer. He inserts a catheter into my uterus, just like he will on transfer day. This allows him to measure the depth of my uterus and determine the best way to insert the catheter during the real transfer. We don't want him overshooting and sending our beautiful embryo(s) somewhere other than my uterus. I'd read about higher IVF success rates with those who had a mock transfer and had meant to ask Dr. Vaughn about it in a previous appointment, but the doc beat me to it. This is why we chose the guy with all the experience.

Chris is traveling, so tonight I have to give myself three shots of Gonal F. Normally it's just one shot, but there wasn't enough of the drugs left in any one Gonal F pen, so I had to take a dose from the three remaining pens. Three times the fun! Luckily I have our cats here to support me. Puck is hanging out on the bathtub (staying away from the alcohol swab) and Tigger is sitting on the counter next to me. Thank you boys, now I don't feel all alone.

I am nervous about giving the shots to myself. But then, how bad can it really be? I take a deep breath and push the plunger in. I should have taken a video of my face to capture the expression. I'm sure it was all scrunched up in anticipation and then a little wince, and then a smile that it was over. Well, at least for shot number one. Two more to go.

***

It's time for another sonogram to check the follicle sizes (the target size is 20mm for IVF). I have nine follicles, many of them in the right range, so Dr. Vaughn says we're ready for the hCG shot tonight and the egg retrieval on Monday. Yeah!

After reading about how painful intramuscular shots can be, I'm a little nervous about Chris giving me my first hCG shot, but if he messes up, I can always try one of the walk-in clinics next time. I'll be taking progesterone shots intramuscularly if I get pregnant, so I'd better just get used to them.

RETRIEVAL DAY

Retrieval day is here. Time to pull those eggs out. During the egg retrieval, I'll be sedated through an IV (oh goodie—more punctures!). The doctor will insert a needle attached to an internal ultrasound probe. The needle will be used to puncture each follicle in combination with a suction that removes the egg and fluid. The embryologist will separate the fluid from the egg and place it together with Chris' sperm in Petri dishes.

Because of the anesthesia, I can't eat or drink after midnight. I guess I will have to hold out on my midnight munchies. No jewelry or nail polish and no contact lenses either, but thankfully I don't need those anymore since the wonders of Lasik (best surgery I ever elected to have).

The alarm brings me out of my subconscious state at 4:45 a.m. so we can be there by 5:15 a.m. for a 6:00 a.m. retrieval. All night, I had a dreadful dream about my alarm not going off and waking up at 10:00 a.m. to find out it's too late and that we've just blown at least half of the IVF fee. That kind of paranoia isn't a recipe for a good night's sleep, not that I expected one anyway.

When we arrive at Austin IVF, the Texas Fertility Center partner for IVF procedures, we are ushered straight into our own room. You can tell this place was just built, as everything's sparkling new. There is a bed, flat screen TV, blood pressure machine, sink and a bathroom. Typical of a hospital but everything looks like it's only just been installed. We are christening the place.

Our nurse, Sunny, is smiling and upbeat—the exact opposite of Chris, who is squinting through his gooey eyes and has already griped two or three times that I am talking too much. I must talk more when I'm nervous, something I've just learned about myself while writing this book.

Sunny asks me if I want the numbing medicine for my IV. I don't know? Seems like a good idea to me. But

Sunny's face says otherwise. I ask her opinion, since she clearly has one. She thinks the numbing medicine is more uncomfortable than the needle itself. So I opt for an IV sans-numbing medicine.

The IV stings like a swarm of bees. Note to self—try the numbing medicine next time.

While we're waiting, Dr. Vaughn pops in to see how we're doing. It's a strange feeling—I've never been this excited to go into "surgery" before. We wait a little longer before Sunny comes back to wheel me down the hall.

Apparently my anesthesiologist, Dr. Mihm (the father of an ex-UT basketball player now NBA player) got lost and was sitting outside of a different building waiting to get in. This is what happens when you're one of the first patients at a brand new clinic. I must say, everything is nice and clean and high-tech though.

Sunny stops the bed in front of the room and has me walk through the doors to the operating room. This is odd. Every other procedure I've had, you're lights out before you get to the operating room. Sunny explains the gurneys from the recovery rooms aren't considered sterile, so that's why they can't wheel it all the way in.

Chris waves goodbye and then heads to his own special room where he'll bottle up his sperm. Apparently, their collection of magazines was far superior in comparison to the clinic where Chris went for testing. Glad he can have fun getting his jollies while I endure a turkey baster jabbing at my insides.

The operating room is freezing cold and I picture my skin being as blue as a Smurf's. They have me wiggle my bottom to the end of the bed, remove my eight-sizes-too-large scrub pants, place my legs in stirrups and splay my arms out to my sides on top of metal wings. This is definitely the most vulnerable position I have ever been in. While I was more excited about this surgery than any other, I feel incredibly uncomfortable, because usually I'm out cold at this point. This time, I'm just cold, not out.

I mention something about being frozen like a Popsicle (we're talking top of a snow covered mountain in your underwear cold), which they may not even understand since my teeth are chattering louder than a jackhammer. Then I add, "I don't think it's going to matter because I definitely feel something warm flowing down my arm." That's the last thing I remember until I wake up in the recovery room with Chris staring down at me.

DR. MIHM

We're both nervous and we have to get up incredibly early. I hate this feeling. My stomach tumbles over like a washing machine from a lack of sleep. I'm sure my nerves are also partly to blame.

It's cold outside; the sun hasn't warmed the gray streets. I'm holding Michelle's hand in the car. The tips of her fingers are chilly. I rub her hand, trying to warm it up.

Once we're all checked in and Michelle is ready to go, our anesthesiologist pads into the room. He's tall as a lumberjack, close to seven feet. He introduces himself as Dr. Mihm.

I smile at the name. Michelle asks him about his son, Chris, a former Longhorn and current NBA player. She loves sports and she wants to hear that the NBA is fun.

He is going on about meeting Phil Jackson, about being in the player family room, and about attending a game in LA. He's telling us about meeting Kobe Bryant. Dr. Mihm is excited to talk about his son. He seems so happy and that is saying something at this time in the morning.

I am glad Michelle likes sports. Not just because it takes her mind off today, but because in some small way, those kids we watch are like our kids. We watch them play. We watch them grow. We watch them learn from their mistakes and succeed. We root for them long after they are gone from campus.

It's time for the retrieval. They're wheeling her into a room for the extraction. I walk her down the hall as far as they will let me, until we arrive at a set of automatic double doors.

I whirl around to find a nurse waiting for me. She asks me if I am ready. From the way she asks me, it feels like she's asking me to go into the Matrix, which would be way more fun than just jerking off in a cup.

I follow her down the hall to the lab. The room has a sink, toilet, a recliner and a drawer of porn—all of the required tools for a successful orgasm in a cup.

She shows me the cup and then a silver door on the wall where I'm to deposit said cup when it's ready.

I can hear the radio on the other side of the door and I can hear someone moving around behind it in the lab. Dark thoughts cross my mind. What would happen if I couldn't perform? This would be a gigantic waste. All the time, money and work and it could all go wrong right here if there aren't any sperm to join Michelle's eggs.

I'm determined not to let that happen.

LESSON 30: FAILURE IS NOT AN OPTION.

DIVIDE, DIVIDE, DIVIDE

The doctor lets us know that he retrieved 11 eggs and that right now, my eggs and Chris' sperm (hopefully they got the labeling right!) are being placed into Petri dishes for conception.

Romantic, isn't it?

I actually don't care how they hook up, as long as they join to form healthy embryos and then divide, divide, divide...

Chris and I talk for an hour while the drugs wear off and then they let me get dressed to go home. I'm to expect a little cramping, which Tylenol should be adequate to quell.

The rest of the day is uneventful. I'm exhausted and go right to bed, which is perfect, since I'm supposed to be resting for 24 hours anyway. Chris heads to work. And he thoughtfully picks up dinner for me on the way home.

That night, Chris has to administer the first <u>progesterone shot</u>. Instead of the suppositories I used for the last two injectables cycles, Dr. Vaughn recommends the shot version instead. After researching online, it sounds like lying down flat on my stomach, with my toes pointed inward, is the safest way to administer the shots correctly. Otherwise, you can hit the sciatic nerve. Definitely don't need that.

Chris is nervous, but does a good job. It hurts like a shot in the arm does, and I rub the area for a while afterwards to try to avoid any painful pockets from forming.

***

The next day, I anxiously call in for our embryo update. Will they say we have almost as many as we did eggs, or will there be two, or one or none and we'll finally have a hint at the reason I haven't gotten pregnant yet?

As usual, I get the clinic's answering machine. Later on, an IVF nurse calls me back to let me know that there are nine fertilized embryos. The conversion rate of eggs to embryos for IVF is typically 70%, so we're above average for once.

The nurse tells me to prepare for a day 3 <u>embryo transfer</u> in two days time, but if there are several good-looking embryos, they'll cancel that morning and reschedule for a day 5 blastocyst transfer.

We're shooting for a day 5 transfer. While a day 3 embryo only has eight cells on average, a <u>blastocyst</u> has 70-100 cells and is just one step away from being ready to implant in the uterine wall. These embryos are also far enough along in development to be graded in several areas.

Several studies I read showed higher success rates with day 5 transfer, which is one reason they typically select only the best two embryos instead of three or more, reducing the chances of multiples. There is a downside though. Some people with plenty of viable embryos at day 3 end up with no embryos to implant by day 5. That would be devastating.

***

On day 3, I set the phone right next to my bed. When the call comes in that there are seven embryos they're watching and that our transfer has been moved to Saturday, I go right back to sleep with a grin planted on my face. In my dreams, I have visions of babies crawling in my head.

Every clinic may use a slightly different grading system, but on day 3, our clinic looks at the following characteristics:

The number of cells (7 cells is the minimum they like to see on day 3).

The Grade (1, 2 or 3). Grade 1 is the best, meaning that all the cells are the same shape and size. Grade 2 embryos show minor imperfections that won't necessarily hinder development. Grade 3 embryos show imperfections that are more likely to prevent proper growth.

<u>Compacting</u> or Not Compacting. Compacting means the embryo shows signs that it is getting ready to turn into a blastocyst. If it is not yet Compacting, that doesn't mean it won't compact, just that it may be a step behind in development.

Chris and I are the proud parents of:

- 2 embryos that are 8-cell, Grade 1, Compacting (our best candidates)
- 2 embryos that are 8-cell, grade 1, not compacting
- 1 embryo that is 7-cell, grade 1, compacting
- 1 embryo that is 8-cell, grade 2, compacting
- 1 embryo that is 7-cell, grade 2, compacting
- 1 4-cell, grade 3, and 1 3-cell, grade 3 (no longer in the running)

THE TRANSFER

It's transfer day and I'm thrilled it doesn't start as early in the morning as retrieval day did. I head over to acupuncture at 9:30 a.m. so they can poke me with a few needles to relax my uterus. Using needles to relax anything sounds counterintuitive to me. Then Chris drives me to the clinic for the <u>embryo transfer</u>.

Sunny's smiling face greets us again. As I change into the clown pants and hospital gown, she hands over a Valium—with the same goal of relaxing my uterus and preventing contractions that can stop the embryo from implanting (I guess the needle-poking wasn't enough). Then she hands me another bottle of water to gulp down. I've already had a bottle the size of a keg on the way over, as instructed. How large do they think my bladder is? I already feel bloated and they expect me to drink another 16 ounces?

Chris has his own gown to put on and he makes a joke about going commando underneath. Thankfully he's all talk. I don't want to see his blinding white butt sticking out the back. He's also jealous of my treaded socks, so he asks Sunny for a pair of his own. She hesitates as if he's just asked her to steal something for him.

I let her know that it's okay—she doesn't need to find him a pair—he can have mine when we're done.

The socks are different though. They're treaded on both sides, which I've never seen before. Sunny explains they moved to the dual sided tread when too many people put them on with the tread-side up (probably my husband included). Now nobody can possibly put them on wrong (unless they try to wear them on another body part, which is something Chris would try).

I'm wheeled down the same hallway as retrieval day and then get off the gurney to walk into the same room, thought it looks completely different. Instead of blinding stadium lights, it's now a cool, extra terrestrial-looking blue.

It's also not nearly as cold this time, and Sunny's taken care to provide extra warmed blankets so that I'm not shaking because what good would relaxing my uterus be if the embryos felt like they'd just entered a volcano?

The embryologist pops in to show us a picture of our two prize embryos. One is a giant compared to the other and definitely looks like a better candidate. Our chances of twins just dropped dramatically.

Dr. Vaughn is busy getting everything ready for the transfer. The embryologist is back in again with a vial suspending the two embryos in fluid. The ultrasound screen is pointed our way so we can watch the procedure. The <u>sono-guided transfer</u> is the reason that my

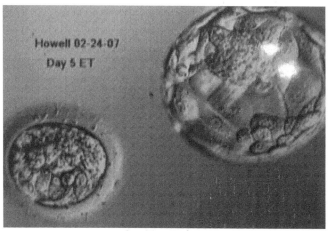

Howell 02-24-07
Day 5 ET

Our Two Embryos

bladder had to be full—it's easier to see the shape of the uterus with my bladder bloated with water.

Having already performed the mock transfer, Dr. Vaughn knows exactly how far to go in—otherwise, the embryo might end up in a fallopian tube, which you definitely do not want. The transfer itself is quick and painless and appears to go smoothly. He snaps a picture of two tiny white dots in my uterus (he has to point them out twice before Chris and I can actually see them) and explains that they're in a great spot just waiting to implant.

Come on you two, attach, attach!

Then the doctor asks me if I think I can make it an hour without relieving my bladder. I don't think I can make it five minutes without exploding. So, he quickly inserts a catheter (I really hate these things) and after a minute, removes it. Ah—bladder relief. I can think about waterfalls without wincing.

Sunny wheels me back to my room and again we're passing the time to wait the painfully long hour, but this time it is much more difficult because although the doctor has emptied my kidney bean bladder, it's already full again. I only make it 45 minutes before I give up. I resist the urge to run and walk calmly to the bathroom. If this IVF doesn't work, I may have my small bladder to blame. Please, please work.

Chris is handed a list of instructions for me, including rest and relaxation, no exercise and pelvic rest for the remainder of the weekend and no alcohol, caffeine, smoking or drugs until the pregnancy test. Damn—I thought I'd be spending the weekend sleeping around and getting wasted.

I stop at the acupuncture clinic for my post-transfer needlework. The acupuncturist tells me they haven't had a miscarriage in the past year, so I'd better not blemish their statistics. I fall asleep in a valium-induced coma and then head home to steal some ZZZZZs.

Now all we can do is wait...

HOPE RESTING ON TWO FLECKS OF LIGHT

I get to stay with Michelle for the transfer procedure. She had to drink 16 ounces of water on our way to the appointment, so she is already uncomfortable.

We're putting in two embryos, which is Dr. Vaughn's recommendation for a day 5 transfer unless we REALLY don't want to have twins. One embryo looks really good and one is a runt in comparison.

I'm dressed in scrubs walking alongside Michelle's bed. We're traversing the white halls into a dark room, glowing blue. I pick the doctor's brain about it.

"It's special lighting because the embryos are sensitive to bright lights," Dr. Vaughn explains.

I thought that it was just to make the room look edgy and cool like a nightclub.

Dr. Vaughn shows us a syringe with a long, snaking rubber tube attached. It's labeled Howell/Miller.

"You will be able to see the embryos on the screen when I insert them," he explains.

Things are going fast at this point. The doctor and nurses are navigating through each step of the process. They speak sparingly but move diligently. They've done this many times before and it shows.

The doctor is using a sonogram machine to guide the embryo transfer. He points to some lighter areas on the screen.

"This is where the cervix is and here is the line of the uterus. I am going to put them right in here."

I'm not at all clear on the orientation of the organs I'm seeing.

"You can see me coming in here."

I see what looks like a tube, coming in from the left.

"I'm going to release it now and you will see two little flecks of light. Three, two, one."

I see a tiny flash of white but I would not know this from a bubble or a glitch with the monitor.

I help Dr. Vaughn and a nurse lift Michelle up and put her on a new gurney. That's when things get weird. The doctors suddenly step back from the gurney with their hands up as if the cart is possessed.

The nurse wheels us into the waiting room. I ask her about the doctors fleeing the scene of the crime. Did I imagine this?

She laughs, and explains, "Doctors believe that it is bad luck to touch the gurney."

Michelle and I laugh at ourselves about our oblivious stares during the sonogram—as usual, we couldn't tell what the hell was going one. Michelle really has to pee, so she tells me not to make her laugh.

"Michelle really has to pee. Can she go?" I ask.

"That's another one of the superstitions. They like you

to wait an hour before moving around. How bad is it?"

Our eyes fall on Michelle.

She looks really uncomfortable.

"I can hold it." She tries to convince herself.

Ten minutes later I have to push the nurse button. Michelle can't hold it any longer. At this point, I hope it's just a superstition, because otherwise we just blew it.

LESSON 31: DOCTORS ARE SUPERSTITIOUS TOO.

THE WAITING GAME

The night of the transfer, I don't want to stress our little embryos, who are hopefully fighting very hard to survive. So we watch the scoreboard of the UT basketball and baseball games instead of watching them live (I get into sports easily, and my heart races when the score is close).

Other than that, we enjoy a relaxing, restful, book-reading and DVD-watching weekend.

One thing that is the sworn enemy of relaxation is the progesterone shot, which Chris has been administering nightly since the day after the embryo retrieval.

My butt is getting sore like a bruised peach with each shot and I am desperate for relief.

I do some research online to see if there are any other tricks to this process. I find many suggestions from women who've been getting the shots for months and test them out—warming the oil in my hand before we put it in the syringe, warming up my butt before the shot, warming the injection site afterwards. Unfortunately, all these are a bust. My rump is still pulsing.

But if I thought the soreness was bad, having a shot come up against a nerve is a thousand times worse. Less than a week after the transfer, I'm ripped from my dreams in the dead of night, a thunderous pain rumbling in my buttocks. It feels like a lightning bolt struck my ass and it's radiating all the way down my right leg.

I clench the aching leg with my hands and lunge it forward, hobbling toward the bathroom. Sleep is out of the question with this stinging pain, and since I could be pregnant, pain medicine is a resounding no. So I head to the family room, start up my laptop and do some research on possible remedies. A heating pad slightly quells the throbbing pain and a few hours later, I'm able to go back to sleep.

I leave a message for the IVF nurse the next morning and she calls back to say I can transition to the progesterone in suppository form instead. I'm hesitant to do this since they obviously have a reason for preferring the shots in the first place, but after more online research, I can't find any proof that one form is more effective than another. Plus, my ass needs a break.

I pick up the progesterone supplements along with the estrogen pills the doctor prescribed. These are apparently only necessary when your estrogen gets really high during IVF, which mine did. Dr. Vaughn explained that I needed to take estrogen supplements to avoid crashing too hard too fast. I guess this way it's a gradual reduction.

***

It's been six days since the transfer and my IVF calendar shows I can call in for our freeze report. I wonder how many of the embryos qualified for freezing. I'm hoping it's several, so we don't have to start from ground zero if this IVF cycle doesn't work.

We can't seem to catch a break.

They weren't able to freeze any of our embryos. Three of the six embryos stopped growing. The other three eventually turned into blastocysts, but didn't meet the stringent criteria. Our clinic used to freeze embryos on day 3, but started to freeze them on day 6 to improve the success rates of frozen embryo transfers. However, as a result, they freeze a lot less of them.

I had a much better feeling about being pregnant until this news. If they didn't make it in a Petri dish, will they really survive and grow inside me?

THE PREGNANT BLOOD

It's been about two weeks since the egg retrieval, and in the funky math of in vitro, this means that the morning has arrived for Michelle to go in for a pregnancy test.

Michelle gets up quietly, trying not to wake me. I can't help it; I wake up anyway. I wish her luck.

When Michelle returns, I ask, "Well did you give them the pregnant blood, or the other stuff?"

She smiles. Then she says, "I really hope I'm pregnant because I feel sick."

"Really?"

"I'm nauseous. But it could just be because I'm nervous," she says.

"You're totally pregnant, because the nausea makes sense. And you smell different."

She brushes this off as my careless optimism.

LESSON 32: SOMETIMES YOU JUST KNOW.

CATCHING OUR FIRST BREAK

It's finally time for my pregnancy test and I am bursting at the seams with nervous energy. My period hasn't started yet, but it could just be a delay as a result of the progesterone shots. I'm nauseous, but that could be nerves.

I get up bright and early to give blood and the results should be available after 1:30 p.m.

I cram my morning full of work to pass the time and then meet Chris for lunch. We call the IVF nurse line on the way back to work and all we get is a busy signal. We try for 20 minutes straight. Unbelievable! We're both fidgety and make small talk for a few minutes before we look at each other and call yet again. I redial at least 30 times while we sit in the car in the parking lot of his office. We finally give up because Chris has to go inside for a conference call. He tells me to keep calling and let him know as soon as I hear something.

ANY NEWS?

I am on calls most of the day. I never call Michelle when I'm at the office. Not for lack of love, but for lack of time. We had lunch together and tried to call the fertility office to no avail.

I call to see if she's heard anything yet. Nothing yet, and I envision her pacing around the room, which is something only I do in our household.

I tell her, "The worst it can be is the same as it was before. Except that you feel like shit and just spent $12,000 for nothing."

So much for lightening the mood. I was just trying to make the worst not seems so bad.

"I have to get on another call, but call me when you know."

LESSON 33: I DON'T ALWAYS SAY THE RIGHT THING.

THE TWO WORDS I'VE BEEN WAITING TO HEAR

I finally get through at around 2:05 p.m.—after 15 rings, an IVF nurse picks up. I can barely get out the words.

Me: "This is Michelle Howell and I'm calling to see if you have the results back from my pregnancy test today."

Nurse: "Hi Michelle. I sure do. We have good news for you."

Me: (My heart pounds and I hope that this woman isn't the type to joke or that there isn't another Michelle and she's mistakenly giving me her results.)

Then she says the two words I've been waiting to hear for more than two years.

Nurse: "You're pregnant. Your numbers look good. Your hCG is 52 and your progesterone is 27. We like to see the hCG between 50-100 at this point, so you're on the lower end."

Me: (Speechless, wondering if I should be thrilled or scared?)

Nurse: "We'll want you to take another blood test in 48 hours to make sure that number goes up and you have a viable pregnancy."

For a few minutes, I debate about going back to Chris' office to tell him in person, but then I worry he'll automatically think something is wrong when he sees me, so I call him instead.

We've told all of the friends and family who we've been updating every step of the way through IVF that the official pregnancy test is tomorrow, so we get to revel in the good news all by ourselves for a day.

SQUIRT

I am on a conference call when our home number pops up on my cell's caller ID. One of my coworkers takes over so I can step out.

I am prepared either way, but I truly believe that it will be good news. Then Michelle says, "As of today I am pregnant. My hCG is at 52 and my progesterone is 27."

After more than two and a half years, countless tests, two surgeries and four fertility treatments, Michelle is finally pregnant. I'm going to be a dad. I feel a tear seep out of the corner of my eye. My hands quiver. I sigh in relief.

Then I remember the numbers she rattled off and realize even being pregnant isn't black and white.

There's still more to worry about. Michelle's hCG number is apparently at the low end of the spectrum for the first test. An auspicious beginning, or nothing to worry about?

Every two days for the next week, Michelle will go in for another blood test to make sure that her hCG number is at least doubling. And they'll watch her progesterone levels to ensure they're high enough to maintain the pregnancy.

When I get home that night, I ask her if she has picked a name. "We are a long way from that," she tells me.

"Not a baby name, but we need to call it something for now. We need a nickname."

She smiles at me. I hope it's one of those smiles where she is secretly admiring my inner child.

"Squirt," I say. "It just fits."

I look down at her belly. "Squirt sure has a long way to go." She laughs. "Squirt." She likes it.

LESSON 34: MAKE EVERY MOMENT COUNT.

FEELING POSITIVE

Later that evening, Dr. Vaughn calls me to say congratulations. He reminds me that it's early, and that we want to see that hCG number at around 80 or more two days from now. But as of today, I am "technically" four weeks pregnant (i.e. it's been four weeks since the first day of my last period and some crazy person decided that would be a good way to measure how pregnant you are).

Even with the news that my hCG number is on the lower end, I feel really positive about this pregnancy. And only as I'm thinking this happy thought does it occur to me that there could actually be more than one. That is a terrifying possibility. But as soon as we started down the fertility path, we knew the chance of getting pregnant with multiples was very high.

THE HAIL MARY

I can't help but smile. It's all turned around. It feels like our backs were against a wall and with a Hail Mary we won the game.

I know this isn't the truth of the matter, as the chances of pregnancy with the first in vitro are around 35%, but it still feels like we beat some long odds.

Even though we have agreed to a full day with the news to ourselves, I'm allowed to tell my brother if he happens to call. My phone rings and it's a weird number, which I know means it's Jake calling from Iraq.

He sounds like he's in a good mood. The last time I spoke with him they were being mortared every night. The airbase was built in a valley, so it was easy for the insurgents to hide in the hills and rain down artillery.

He tells me things are better, the mortaring only happens about once a week and the accuracy has dropped significantly. The Marines now respond so quickly they only get off a couple of rounds, and then they've eliminated the threat.

I finally get a chance to tell him the good news and I can hear he's smiling in his voice, even though the connection is bad and spans so many thousands of miles.

In his voice I can tell he appreciates the journey we've been through. He tells me to pass along congratulations to Michelle.

He asks me if we have a name. I explain that we really haven't let it sink in, but share our nickname for now.

We reminisce about moments in our childhood. He reminds me that I used to kidnap him, under the auspice of taking him to eat, and then lecture him on life. I know it's true. And I know he's warning me about the impact some of my antics would have on my child.

For once, we actually get to talk for about an hour, instead of getting disconnected after 10 minutes. I need to remember to pay him back for the call. It's not expensive but he makes so little, every bit is material.

We hang up and I can't help but smile. He's doing well and he's going to be an uncle someday. I relish the thought of my children playing with Uncle Jake. Even Dr. Seuss wrote about it in *Oh, the Places You'll Go!*

LESSON 35: LITTLE BROTHERS CAN TEACH THEIR BIG BROTHERS LESSONS TOO.

SPREADING THE GOOD NEWS

The next day, I send out the following email to our clan:

Well, as of today, I'm four weeks (and one day) pregnant. Obviously it's VERY EARLY and there's up to a 25% chance that things can take a turn between now and the magical 12-13 week mark, but since we've been sending you all of the IVF updates, we thought you'd want to hear the news.

My hCG level was on the lower end of the spectrum (it was 52 and they like it to be between 50-100), but what apparently matters most is not the actual number but that the number doubles every 48 hours.

I'll have another blood test this week to check that things are still progressing normally. If all goes well with the blood tests, we'll have our first sonogram to listen for the baby's heartbeat (or multiple heartbeats if there are two!) in about three weeks. We'll keep you posted...

Thank you for all of your support, finger/toe crossings and prayers!

Love,

Michelle & Chris

Two days later, I go in for my next blood test and we hear great news. My hCG is 113—more than double, my progesterone is 31, and my estradiol is 464—all normal. The hCG number should double every 48-96 hours, depending on where you are in the pregnancy. A guideline is when the hCG is less than 1,200, it should double every 48-72 hours. When it's between 1,200-6,000, it slows down to doubling every 72-96 hours. And when it's above 6,000, it will only double every 96 hours until the hCG hormone is no longer increasing (about the end of the first trimester).

I have my first visit to the grocery store as a pregnant woman. No deli meats? What am I going to eat for lunch? And I guess I shouldn't wash it all down with a soda and a package of Oreos. Do I really have to avoid edamame and all things soy? And almost every bottle of salad dressing appears to have eggs in the ingredients. Does that mean I can't eat dressing at all? So many questions...

Of course, I didn't come this far to screw things up now, so I'll stick to the rules.

I thought the wait between the first few blood tests was tough, but now they're scheduled for once a week. I swear it's been much longer than a week and I'm only on day 4. Day 7 finally rolls around and I'm anxiously waiting to hear the magic numbers.

I'm on my way to lunch with my very pregnant sister and two nieces when I get the call. I sit down on a wall outside Central Market and whip out my notepad before picking up the call. My heart has crept past my throat and across the street. It's galloping as fast as a racehorse. I don't know why I'm so nervous, but it must be the prospect of coming this far and then losing it all.

The nurse says my numbers still look good and I let out a sigh of relief. My hCG is up to 1,300 and the progesterone and estradiol numbers are within normal range. The nurse instructs me to keep taking the progesterone supplements, to take two more days of the estrogen pills, and then check in for another blood test next week.

The news warms my heart, which has finally slowed to a horse's trot. It's a beautiful, sunny day in Austin. And having lunch with my family is icing on the cake.

TJ

Chris is stuck at work and with all our IVF appointments over and the waiting game just beginning, I decide to get out in the sun. So I snatch my laptop and head off to a UT baseball game, planning to get a little work done while cheering on our Longhorns.

A few innings into the game, I realize there's a 6-year-old boy staring over my shoulder from the row behind me. Actually, I may not have noticed him except I catch a whiff of his sumptuous hot dog. My stomach grumbles like a beast.

Within a few minutes, TJ and I are fast friends. He leans over my lap to see my computer screen and asks me to go to his favorite websites so he can play games (which I can't do, since you need a UT access code). So we find other ways to entertain ourselves. We enter his birthday in my calendar, which happens to be my "due date"—November 14th. I smile and look down at my tummy.

TJ is a little chatterbox. I teach him how to read the scoreboard. TJ's mom checks in to make sure I'm okay with this arrangement and I assure her I am.

TJ isn't that interested in the game. He mostly cares about seeing his cousin, who plays for Stanford, come out on the field. He and his mom had driven in from Dallas to watch him play. Unfortunately, his cousin isn't a starter for the team yet, so TJ waits patiently until he finally comes in to pinch-hit.

I can honestly say it was one of the best baseball games I've ever been to, and it was all because of the company (no offense Chris). We ask one of the Stanford kids for a ball and TJ grins from ear to ear when the player plops it in his eager hands. We cheer while his cousin hits a triple (well, TJ cheered—I couldn't betray the Horns, but I was happy to see the guy get a hit and score a run for TJ's sake). Stanford makes a ninth-inning push, but UT finally closes it out and while the crowd sings "The Eyes of Texas," TJ and I sadly say our goodbyes.

It's going to sound corny, but I felt like the day was a sign. All of those questions about whether we were doing the right thing—if it was worth all the heartache and grief and pain and money. Should we, in a sense, play God by undergoing fertility treatments that spit out ten times the amount of eggs my body would normally release in a month or try to conceive a child in a Petri dish? Maybe we just aren't meant to have children. But after a day with TJ, I gain a calm sense of reassurance that it is in the cards. And the lively little boy is my sign of what I have to look forward to.

Chris and I are on walk that night and he says, "I sure hope nothing goes wrong with Squirt, because I'd be crushed."

I know what he means. While we would normally be optimistic, we remain reserved until I've made it to the second trimester. But it does feel like everything is finally going right for us.

GLOWING

I am in awe. That there is a part of us, Squirt, growing inside Michelle is incredible. Squirt is doing masterful work. Michelle is glowing.

This isn't the first time she's glowed. When I proposed, I think that there was a bit of a shimmer, a hint of an aura surrounding her. When I tickle her and when she is incredibly happy, she glows. (It's a magical glow, not a scary alien kind of thing). Also perhaps I've seen her look this way when we were at Disney World, the time I begged her to ride the Tower of Terror three times in a row, or when I paid her $1,000 to jump into a cold pool and swim with me.

But all of those glows are but a faint and pale illumination compared to this.

We go for a walk, making sure not to walk too fast. We chat about Squirt, about the journey so far, about the journey ahead. I comment on how much great material there is for this book. We've been through trying on our own, IUI, injectables, acupuncture and in vitro.

Michelle's breasts are already swollen. Thank you Squirt! Unfortunately, they also quite sensitive (Squirt help me out here), which makes my enjoyment mainly visual.

The blood tests are down to once a week, with the next one coming up in two days. Her nausea has subsided the last couple of days and she is anxious about the next test.

**

In the morning, I leave for a conference in Dallas. I promise to call her when I get finished with my day. I pat Squirt and remind him or her to be good and say goodbye.

LESSON 36: ENJOY THE JOURNEY.

PART IV

HEAVEN AND EARTH

A BAD DREAM

My nausea has subsided a bit, and Tigger, who had reli-
giously slept against my belly for the last two weeks,
hasn't come into bed to cuddle the last few nights.
When the alarm goes off for my weekly blood test,
I find myself alone in bed. That's when I remember
Chris is out of town.

I make a mental note to schedule our heartbeat
sonogram when the nurse calls with the test results. I
can't wait to see our baby and hear the heartbeat (or
more than one heartbeat, which is still a possibility,
though they say your hCG numbers are usually higher
with twins and mine appear to be in the normal range).

Usually, the nurse calls by around 2:00 p.m., so

when I don't hear anything by 3:00 p.m., I call the IVF line and leave a message. I have some light cramps today—definitely a different feeling than anything I've had up until this point. Is it just the pregnancy—my uterus starting to stretch? Or is it more ominous than that? Combined with the nausea change, an unsettling feeling creeps into my bones by the hour.

The fertility clinic closes at 4:00 p.m. and when that time comes with no word, I accept the fact that I'm not getting the results today.

I call Chris and he tells me not to worry.

I try not to worry, but I know that one third of all first pregnancies miscarry. This statistic seems high to most people because you rarely hear stories about miscarriages until you have one yourself or have a friend or relative go through one. I read online that OBs usually won't talk about the statistics of miscarriages because pregnancy is supposed to be a positive, happy occasion. All of my research is fuel to my anxiety fire.

That night, I dream that the nurse calls to let me know my hCG levels don't look good—that they haven't doubled. She says in an ominous, echoing voice, "I'm sorry." I wake up from my nightmare in a cold sweat.

Since Chris is traveling, I have nobody but the kitties to comfort me. Tigger must sense that I need some loving, because he comes in a few minutes later to sleep across my legs.

It takes me hours to fall back to sleep. My mind rolls through all of the reasons the nurse wouldn't have called with the results. The fear and anxiety of the worst possibility slowly crawls under my skin and wraps me in its clutches. And for the first time, it hits me that I could, at this very moment, no longer be pregnant.

ON THE WRONG SIDE OF THE STATISTICAL WAR

I've been calling the IVF line all morning and leaving a message maybe once for every four tries. No response. I try several times in the afternoon. Doesn't anyone ever answer the *@&$!%#$ phone?

I imagine myself driving down to the clinic, barging through the door, grabbing my chart and reading it myself. If someone tries to stop me, I'll say, "Then answer your damn phone next time!"

I call one more time at 3:50 p.m. (the office closes at 4:00 p.m.) and leave this message in the nicest tone I can:

"This is Michelle Howell again. I apologize for leaving several messages today, but I'm getting a little nervous that the lack of response means something is wrong. If for some reason you don't have the results of my blood test yesterday, please call me and let me know that. I just need to know something, as I'm going a little crazy waiting for a response."

I also make a last-ditch effort by calling the regular nurse line to see if they can track down the information for me, but I get their answering machine as well.

No news is not likely good news, and I have a lump in my throat the size of lemon (I think it was more comfortable when the lemons were in my ovaries).

Tigger is roaming around the house crying and I can't figure out what's wrong with him. Maybe he knows something I don't. He still hasn't come to cuddle up next to my belly.

I call Chris to see if he thinks I should go watch the baseball game by myself when the other line beeps. I tell Chris I'll call him back and click over with dread.

I stop my pacing and sit down on the floor. My vision has gone blurry.

The nurse apologizes for the delay in getting back to me. Things have been crazy. She'd been waiting for the doctor to review the test results. Yadda, yadda, yadda.

Lady, give me the news already!

Then she grants my wish. Except then, I wish she hadn't.

Just like my nightmare, I get a swift slap in the face from reality. The nurse tells me my hCG number has barely doubled in a week's time. It is only 2,348 and it should be closer to 10,000 by now.

She explains, "That is not an appropriate rise. The doctor's afraid that this hCG level indicates it is not a good pregnancy. We'd like you to take another blood test tomorrow morning in case there was a mistake and then come in for a sonogram tomorrow afternoon."

My brain reverts to autopilot. I mechanically schedule the sonogram. I'm numb and the whole world seems to be floating in slow motion around me.

After I hang up, the numbness gives way to anger. Are you fucking kidding me? Why can't anything be easy? Haven't we given enough already?

SHIT. SHIT. SHIT.

Then the denial creeps in. Maybe the test results were wrong? But I have light cramps and no nausea and everything points to the fact that this baby is no longer developing.

I call Chris back and tell him the bad news. He is quiet for a moment. Then he sighs and whispers, "Oh, Squirt."

My eyes water and my heart aches.

Still in a hushed tone, he asks, "Do you want me to drive back to Austin tonight?"

My throat twists and burns, signs of the tears that are bubbling up in my soul. The tears finally escape and I can barely breathe.

Chris then starts on all of the things we could have done wrong. We've been walking more lately—maybe I overdid it.

I want to scream, "Stop it!" but I don't have the strength. The fact that I'm miscarrying is bad enough, but to tell me it's directly my fault and could have been avoided is more than I can take.

If he was in front of me, I'd probably punch him in

the gut.

Or kick him in the shin.

Or throw him out the window.

Throwing something sounds like a great idea. I throw a pillow. Then another. That's not doing it for me. I decide tearing up the pillows would be much more satisfying. I'm lying in the middle of my bed surrounded by shredded pillows, watching a feather float down toward my face.

"Michelle?" Chris asks hesitantly, breaking me out of my feather-riddled fantasy. I look around to see our perfectly made bed.

Always the optimist, Chris says, "Look at it this way. Now we have another chapter for our book."

This actually makes me laugh. The good kind of laugh that releases some of my pent up emotion.

He has a good point. Now we can cover just about every possible infertility hurdle. Not getting pregnant on our own. Not getting pregnant with stimulation drugs. Getting pregnant with our first IVF and then having a miscarriage. I only hope we eventually have content for a happy ending chapter where I get pregnant and have a healthy child!

I know it's only because I'm partially in denial that I can think positively. There's still a piece of me that hasn't accepted reality. There's still hope until I see the doctor tomorrow.

It's 15 minutes before the first pitch. We say goodbye so I can go to the game and Chris can go work out.

The tears stream down my face as I walk out the door.

DEVASTATING NEWS

The nurse finally called Michelle back and said that the test results aren't looking good. Her hCG number should be higher.

I'm crushed.

I'm devastated for Michelle.

I have never felt more powerless.

I miss Squirt.

I offer to drive back to Austin and then drive back to Dallas for my meeting the following morning—if only just to cuddle and hold her in my arms. Michelle lets me off the hook.

I try to stay cheerful on the phone. I remind her that things always work out for the best. We are strong and we can make it through anything together.

I hope I'm right.

I struggle to think of any positive spin I can put on this.

I call Michelle back and offer up the only hope I can. "We can try fertility treatments as many times as it takes." And I mean it. I'll do whatever I need to, to make this possible.

Michelle seems to appreciate this. Her voice seems a little lighter, with a bit of hope mixed in with the pain. Or so I want to believe.

I know we still have a long healing process to go through.

Squirt is gone, and there is a gaping hole in my heart.

LESSON 37: SOMETIMES LIFE HURTS UNIMAGINABLY.

PREPARING FOR THE INEVITABLE

Chris calls back minutes later and says we can try IVF as many times as it takes. I'm touched, because that says a lot. Initially, he wanted me to agree to only one or two tries and eventually we settled on three.

My family is waiting to hear the results of the latest blood test, but I'm not ready to tell anyone else yet because I don't have all the facts. And I'm also not prepared to deal with them trying to comfort me. Besides, what if I tell them about the hCG results and then some miracle happens and there's still a healthy baby growing inside of me? I stall—shooting off a brief email that I need to take another blood test in the morning.

On my way to the baseball game, there is someone I do want to talk to. I call my friend Jennifer, who had a miscarriage on her first try. I want to know what to expect when I go to the sonogram tomorrow. And what to expect after the confirmation is made. I get her voicemail.

I'd been hesitant about going to the game, but it's a good distraction. I tell myself I can't handle UT losing, so if the team isn't playing well, I'll just have to leave. But luckily Texas holds on to win 5-3.

I'm relieved that our baseball friends Marc and Barbara aren't there, because they know I'm pregnant and they surely would have said something about the baby that is probably no longer alive inside me. I would have turned into a flowing fire hydrant again.

The only bright side I can think of is that as early as tomorrow afternoon, I can stuff my face with jellybeans and candy corns. I guess my raging sweet tooth is the only thing that wins in this situation.

When I return home, I research online to see if it's at all possible to not double your hCG count in a week and still have a healthy baby. It doesn't look good. And it sounds like there's a possibility the pregnancy could be <u>ectopic</u> (outside the uterus), which could require surgery. Will this saga ever end? Sometimes the Internet is not my friend.

I also research what tests should be done to determine the cause. More than 70% of the time, miscarriages are a result of a genetic defect in the embryo. If possible, I definitely want to know the cause, because there is a list of other reasons that are problems with the "host" (a.k.a. ME!) and I'd sure like to know if that's the case before going through another IVF cycle.

I get in bed around 11:00 p.m. but read a book until I've finished it—until about 1:00 a.m.—so that I don't have the energy to outthink sleep. I can feel the cramps grinding at my insides. And suddenly a new wave of despair sweeps over me. For the first time, I feel like giving up.

Maybe it just isn't meant to be. It feels like my whole reality is crumbling beneath the weight of this one incident. I've lived and breathed creating a baby for 30 months, and now it all ends with a single defective embryo. I don't know how women who suffer through multiple miscarriages continue to try. Especially those who have to go through the hassle of fertility drugs first. I just can't imagine the strength that must take. I curl up in a ball like a toddler, and hug my pillow.

THE WORST DAY

My alarm is incessantly buzzing and while I want to hurl it across the room, I resist the urge, mostly because I know it is pretty resilient and will likely continue its annoying buzz until I get up and turn it off.

My eyes well up with tears as I pet Puck good morning.

I brush my teeth, get dressed and drive to the lab all in a dazed state.

As I'm getting my blood drawn, I ask the technician how often the lab makes mistakes.

"Never," she replies.

Thanks for giving me hope! I yell, "Have any dreams you'd like me to crush?" as I pull the needle from my arm and throw it like a dart across the room. It hits a poster, right between the eyes of a mother holding hands with her two small children.

I'm forced back to reality when she says, "I'm all done," gently removing the needle and labeling the vial of blood.

And that's what I feel like—all done.

At least this is probably the last blood test I'll have for a while.

There is still a tiny part of me that thinks there could have been a mistake. I'm sure that's what people often think when they're told a loved one has died. If you don't see it with your own eyes, it's so hard to accept something you don't want to believe.

Whenever I feel down, I watch the movie *The Little Mermaid*. I haven't watched it in several years, but I think it's time to pop that DVD in.

Maybe I should save the movie. I'll probably be much sadder then than I am now. Though that's hard for me to imagine.

What I'm dreading most of all is the family calls I'll have to make after I get the official word. I could send everyone an email and tell them I'm not up for talking, but that would make them upset and worried instead of just upset. I suppose it's a positive sign that I can still think about the feelings of others. Though I just want to crawl in a dark hole and block out the world.

While the clock ticks along slowly, I get online to check my email. There's one from a childhood friend, saying: A little birdie told me that congratulations are in order! Woohooo! I know it's still early, but I wanted to let you know I'm thinking of you and Chris and so excited for the new addition(s?)!

My throat closes up and I fight away the tears.

It is really no wonder that everyone recommends not sharing the news until after you're past the first trimester. I don't mind that people know, and that now they'll know I've had a miscarriage. But it would be better for them and easier for me if only my spouse and I were dealing with the news.

But hey, I got pregnant, which is a good sign even if I am having a miscarriage. A friend's fertility doctor had made this exact comment to her after her first miscarriage and she was so annoyed with his aloofness that she switched doctors. But his point remains true—that is a big hurdle.

I know I can get pregnant. Now I just have to figure out how to get pregnant and stay pregnant.

I continue to drift through the day in a trance, barely paying attention to the world around me. It's a miracle I don't get in a car accident on the way to the fertility clinic.

I make the mistake of going to the doctor's appointment by myself instead of taking a friend along. I thought that if Chris couldn't come with me, it would be easier to handle alone. And I didn't want to dump my sadness on an innocent bystander. There was still a chance they got it wrong, right?

Usually all smiles, Dr. Vaughn enters the room with a solemn expression. I can tell I am doomed before he utters the tragic words, "I'm sorry."

I reply, "I was hoping the next time I saw you it would be for a happy heartbeat sonogram." I try to smile but my facial muscles don't cooperate.

He tells me my hCG count has gone down again since Monday. Now I am just praying that the embryo is in the right place so that I might be able to have a child in the future.

My prayer is answered—the yolk sac is right in the middle of my uterus.

If there is a heaven, I hope little Squirt's soul is there now.

I am afraid to look at the screen because I don't want the picture of my dead fetus to haunt me for the rest of my life. But I can't resist a peek. I'm drawn to it like all of the stupid rubberneckers I swear at. But when I do take a peek, there isn't much to see.

Dr. Vaughn can clearly see I'm distraught, which is probably why he doesn't mention I have a <u>blighted ovum</u> (an empty sac with no embryo). I am too out of it to ask more questions. That's probably a good thing.

Dr. Vaughn explains that since I'm not very far along, I can just let my body expunge the embryo on its own instead of having a <u>D&C</u>. But if it starts to drive me crazy, he can take care of it right away. I should stop taking the progesterone and expect cramps and heavy bleeding in the next week.

Wash away the old and start with the new.

While I don't feel present in the room, I hear myself ask him when we can try another in vitro cycle. I'll have to wait until one month after my hCG level returns to zero. I was very wrong about this morning's blood test being the last one for a while. I'll need to go once a week to check my hCG level. I'll stab the nurse then.

I also ask if we should do any testing to find out why this happened. Dr. Vaughn says it's just a genetic defect in the embryo—that there's probably nothing else to learn.

The tears start to cloud my eyes and the he says, "Take all the time you need," before leaving me alone in the room. As soon as the door closes I break down into sobs. Once I regain control and find some tissues, I call Chris and tell him the news.

Chris made me simultaneously laugh and cry when I receive an email reply from his BlackBerry seconds later that says, "I miss Squirt already." I touch my belly, tears streaming down my face. I miss Squirt too.

THANKS FOR THE HOPE SQUIRT

It's late in the afternoon and I see Michelle calling me. I pick it up and immediately sense the anguish in her voice. Our worst fears have been confirmed. She's not crying but I can hear the tears welling up, ready to burst. Dr. Vaughn has just walked out of her exam room and she is sitting there alone. The baby is no longer growing. Squirt is no more.

I'm in my hotel room, staring at a painting of a horse in the distance, standing on a snow-covered hill all alone. I hate this picture, maybe because it reminds me of how I feel. Alone.

Did I mention that this process can completely and totally suck? This is painful. I miss Squirt. I miss the feeling of knowing something is growing. It's the end after such a short beginning. I miss knowing that we will have a child someday.

But right now, those are selfish thoughts, because I need to focus on Michelle. She's been pretty resilient up until now. This could be her breaking point.

The doctor has advised her that there are things she can do to help the miscarriage along, or she can just wait it out. I would like to say that this means that it could still reverse, but that is not the case. It's awful that we have to think about these options at this time. But just like everything in this process, the timing does matter.

I'm angry and frustrated because I am in a hotel in Dallas, not with Michelle. I'm finding an earlier flight tomorrow.

Most of all, my heart aches. My body shutters. The emotional distress has manifested itself in the form of sheer physical pain. Nothing any client says means anything to me on this day. I hear them, I respond, I may even laugh, but behind my eyes the lights are out.

I'm sorry we failed you Squirt. I'm choked up about what might have been. After all, he or she is the only kid I almost had.

I call Michelle multiple times that night and the next day, making sure to let her talk it out. I also want and need to hear her voice. I keep her positive; there will be a next time. I want to make sure she has hope to counter the feeling of loss.

We'd agreed to try in vitro only three times. But I remind her we can try as many times as she wants. "I'll borrow money, get a different job or do whatever it takes. We can make this all work. I won't give up."

Then I say, "There is good news." I pause for dramatic effect and to make sure that she is listening. "You can get pregnant. We know that now. It's just a few more steps."

And it really is positive news. Michelle was pregnant. So something is working right and this is farther than we've ever been before. So on the bright side, I look up to the sky and say thank you to Squirt. Thanks for the hope.

LESSON 38: NEVER, EVER GIVE UP.

SHARING THE BAD NEWS

When I get home from the fertility office, I send the following email to the family and friends who'd been getting IVF updates:

I wish I was writing with better news, but our little embryo stopped growing last week, which was confirmed by two hCG blood tests (Monday morning and this morning) and a sonogram about an hour ago. More than 70% of first trimester miscarriages are a result of one or more genetic defects, and this appears to be the culprit in our circumstance. The doctor said there's no way to know if it was my genes or Chris' genes, but Chris said he'd take the blame.

The bright side is that I can get pregnant (actually a giant hurdle for the fertility-challenged), that the embryo implanted in the right place and that my hormone levels appear to be able to sustain a pregnancy just fine.

And to Chris' point, it's also another chapter for our He Said/She Said Fertility Book—I think we've covered just about everything as long as we have a healthy baby some day!

Thank you all for your good wishes, love and support. Love, Michelle

I call my parents so that they hear the news from me instead of my email.

Me: "Hi. Well, I just sent you an email update, but I wanted to call and let you know our little embryo stopped growing."

Mom: "Oh no. Oh Michelle, I'm so sorry."

Dad: "I thought there were two?"

Mom: "No Ladd, there is only one."

Dad: "But I thought there were two embryos."

Mom: "Ladd!" (i.e. Stop Talking!)

Mom: "Oh Michelle, I'm so sorry." (This is a line she would repeat at least five more times before I got off the phone.)

Dad: "So what happens now?"

Me: "Well, I'm not far along enough to need a D&C, so I think I'm going to let my body try to handle it on its own. If I run into any problems, or if I get impatient, the doctor said I just needed to call and he'd do a D&C for me."

Mom: "You know a D&C can actually increase your chance of getting pregnant. I had a D&C four years ago—well no, it had to have been more than four years ago because I could still get pregnant—and the doctor warned me that the D&C could increase my chances of getting pregnant, so I needed to be careful. So if you do have to have a D&C, there might be a positive in that."

Me: "Hmmm. I hadn't heard that. I'll have to do some research on it."

Mom: "Can we come see you and give you a big hug?" (i.e. Do you want us to get on a plane from Florida?)

Me: "No—that's okay. I'll see you when you come for Sarah's surgery in April."

My four-year-old niece is having open-heart surgery in a month and we'll all be in Houston for that. It's a good reminder that I still have so much to be thankful for, even at a time like this.

Mom: "We love you."

Miraculously, I manage to get off the call without shedding a tear.

But the call with my sister does not go quite as smoothly. She hits my heart about ten minutes into the call with the question, "How are you feeling?" I get out the words, "Emotionally or physically?" before I break down.

My tears sting with pain and disappointment, prompting her to cry with me. She volunteers to come see me tomorrow, or even tonight if I need her to. A day at the spa? I suggest we plan to meet up some time next week. Hopefully, I'll have stopped randomly sobbing by then.

Laura calls back an hour later to offer us two Southwest tickets to get away. "I thought maybe you'd want to go somewhere, like Las Vegas or San Diego or Orlando. You could go anywhere..."

I thank her and let her know that I'll talk to Chris

about it.

Then I flop down on the couch to enjoy my jellybeans and candy corns (for candy corn lovers, the Brachs pastel candy corn bag at Easter is the best!). Chris asks me if he is going to come home from the airport to have dinner and look across the table to see a plate of candy in front of me as my meal. When I realize that I can barely taste the sugar, I stop eating it.

My mother-in-law calls me later that night to see how I'm doing and to tell me she loves me. She asks if there is anything she can do just for me. I promise to think about it and let her know.

Chris comes home and cuddles with me and I can feel some of my sadness dissipate. He is my prince charming. My best friend. My safety net. And as his arms wrap around me, the pent up tension in my head and neck and shoulders and stomach finally releases. I go limp like a dead eel.

***

The next day, my email inbox is brimming with replies of sympathy and phone calls from my mom and sister to make sure I haven't jumped off a bridge or gone stark, raving mad. I tell them not to worry—I've locked up all the guns.

Two cookie bouquets arrive that afternoon. Tigger sniffs around the Tigger-shaped cookies that I'm convinced he'll have no interest in. I break off an ear anyway and put it on the counter for him to smell. Clearly, I was wrong. He licks it a couple times, then gulps down the whole piece. I guess now I'll have to find a safe place to store them away from the cats.

THE LOADED QUESTION

I've noticed that I am not myself lately. I'm sure I am grumpy, I am careful around Michelle and I generally don't want to talk to anyone. I certainly don't want to answer the phone when it rings. But I check the number and it's some non-descript impossibly long series of digits, which means it is nearly certain to be my brother.

Within the first few seconds, I can tell Jake doesn't know, so I tell him about the miscarriage.

"Well you're going to try again, aren't you?" he asks.

There is no hesitation in the question, no polite silence, he just asks. And this chokes me up.

I draw in a long deep breath, stabilizing myself and say, "Yes."

And somehow this makes me feel better. I'm not sure if it is my answer or his question.

Maybe it's because the last time we spoke, he told

me about a pilot in his squadron whose corpse was paraded through the streets by the Taliban and televised on CNN. I'm reminded about how lucky I am, even when I don't feel lucky at all.

Or maybe it's because I can hear the concern in his voice. He wants to know if I still have hope. He's asking the loaded question.

Inside I am churning. I feel spent. Do I have hope? In truth I am full of doubt. My focus is on keeping Michelle happy, but do I believe anymore?

I am always the guy who has hope. I guess I normally have a bit more confidence. I believe anything is possible. And I am a bit of a gambler. In the past when I didn't have hope, I could fake it and push myself through it.

Asking the very question steels my resolve. Jake asking the question bolsters it. I can think of no other option; I must have hope and so somehow suddenly, I do.

I think it is because for so long he was my little brother. I've had to give him hope, or at least I thought I should. But maybe the whole time it was exactly as it is today. By reassuring him, I am reassuring myself.

My brother reminds me so much of my grandfather. It's too bad the two of them didn't get to spend more time together when Jake was older. They would have argued like hell and loved every minute of it.

After my answer we talk about other things; anything but the miscarriage. We have a great relationship and seem to know what to say to each other in times like these.

Suddenly, he says he has to go, and before I can even say goodbye the line goes dead. I get to worry about him along with everything else.

LESSON 39: GETTING OLDER SUCKS. I WANT TO BE A KID AGAIN.

WHAT DO WE DO NOW?

The thought of having a miscarriage in the middle of a grocery store, or waiting and waiting for the miscarriage to happen only to have it drag on are now my two biggest concerns. The decision not to have a D&C became easier because my insurance restarts on January 1, not April 1 like I thought. So the idea of spending $2K on my deductible doesn't sound very appealing, especially since even if I get pregnant on our next IVF try, I won't be delivering until 2008.

Laura had mentioned a third option—<u>Misoprostol</u>—a pill that's supposed to move the miscarriage process along. My fertility clinic doesn't offer this, so I call my regular OB/GYN and leave a message for her nurse to see what she recommends. Then I head back to the kitchen for a Tigger cookie and a large glass of milk. I catch Tigger working his way through the packaging for another bite of cookie. I give him a small piece; at least the cat can get what he wants. My OB's nurse calls back a few hours later and schedules me for an appointment the next day.

***

Dr. Gunter tells me a story of a patient who waited more than four weeks for her miscarriage to occur. I just want to get this whole thing over with as soon as possible. I'll take the first pill on Sunday night and then if nothing happens, I'm to take another one on Monday night. If that doesn't work, she can do a D&C Tuesday afternoon or Wednesday morning (I figured if I did end up needing the D&C, she had to have more of these under her belt than my fertility doctor did).

She describes what I should look for in the form of tissue to save and deliver to their office to make sure the miscarriage is complete. I'm not looking forward to acting like Hannibal Lecter and collecting it.

When I get home from the doctor's office, I look through forum after forum to make sure my plan is actually the right decision. After a lot of research, I'm not completely convinced the Misoprostol route is the right one. Though I doubt I'll be 100% comfortable with any of the options no matter how much information I have on them. I still have this irrational fear that the baby is possibly alive and I'd be killing it. I tell myself to cut it out. Myself finally listens.

I drag my listless body to the bathtub and soak in the scorching water. The hot water opens up my pores and brings to the surface a deep sadness. Most of the day I've been avoiding touching the true depth of my hurt. But the stillness of the water combined with my undivided attention brings me to the edge. I have never known loss like this before. It is such a raw ache in my soul that it brings uncontrollable sobs. I guess it is best to meet my pain in person, shake its hand and chat with it like old friends.

A few minutes past midnight, I ask Chris to talk me into taking the pill—it's the only way I'm going to be able to get over the indecision hump. I wrap myself under the covers and within thirty minutes, I feel the cramping start. Chills spread like tentacles from my head to my toes. I endure the night after taking a Naproxen for the cramps and thinking about all of my favorite vacations.

The next morning, there appears to be tissue the size of a Q-tip, along with a few blood clots. I drop off the sample and head straight back home. My subsequent stomach issues cause me to visit the bathroom frequently, a warned side effect of the pill (especially when taken orally).

The OB's office calls to tell me they aren't sure that's all there is, so I'm instructed to take another Misoprostol tonight. Shit—the cramps were finally subsiding.

I do a lot of research on Naproxen this time in case that's what prevented the Misoprostol from working. I don't find sufficient evidence that it's okay, even though both doctors said it was, so I take a Tylenol 3 with Codeine instead. That bugger doesn't work nearly as well and I'm up until three in the morning with chills and cramps.

There is much more bleeding and blood clots and cramps the next day. These cramps are definitely different than the usual monthly variety. They hit me like a linebacker—strong, quick and then subside, only to start over again thirty minutes later. Not the constant, dull ache I'm used to on the first day of my period.

My mom almost passes out when she hears I could be cramping and bleeding for another two weeks, saying, "Oh God, I thought it was almost over!"

Nope. It seems like it is never over with this circus act we call infertility.

I do find an article that adequately explains why Naproxen does not impact the effectiveness of Misoprostol and a research study that shows no significant impact between the Naproxen group and a control group. So I take a Naproxen 30 minutes before heading to a baseball game. It kicks in an hour later.

My acupuncturist stimulates some of the needles with electricity to help the miscarriage process along (as if the feeling of the needles wasn't creepy enough) and provides me with herbs to do the same. I tell them I'm sorry I messed up their statistics.

The bleeding finally stops four days later, but the heartache takes much longer to heal. It feels as though a light that's always burned strong inside of me has been snuffed out and I don't know how to turn it on again.

A LONG WAY TOWARD HEALING

I finally have to tell my mom and sister to stop using THE VOICE every time I talk to them. You know, the somber tone that sounds like they're worried you're about to slit your wrists. Every conversation invariably begins with a soft-spoken, "How are you?" I resist the urge to respond, "I feel like shit. How are you?"

My hCG levels drop from 2,200 to 215 to 14 to 2 and then finally to zero. I read that it could take months to get to zero, so I consider myself lucky. Trying to think positively, I'm also happy to be done with the blood tests for a while.

At my OB check-up, the doctor says everything looks good and notes that I'm cleared for sexual activity. Good thing, because I didn't know that was a restriction and we'd already jumped back on that boat a few nights ago.

***

My sister and nieces are in town to cheer me up. Sarah, the oldest, is four, and was born with a heart condition that she already had open-heart surgery to repair before she was a year old. Now a new issue has come up and she's scheduled for another surgery in two weeks. Everything has to go well. I plainly explain to God that he can't take two family members in this short period of time.

It's my two-year-old niece, Reese, who makes me realize that I've begun to recover from my loss. Since Laura is pregnant and they knew I was too, whenever I'd come visit, Reese would capture my heart with those big beautiful brown eyes and say, "You have a baby in your belly." We're sitting in the kitchen eating a bowl of ice cream when Reese looks up at me, this time with sad eyes and says, "Michelle, you don't have a baby in your belly anymore."

Two weeks ago, that might have sent me into an uncontrollable sobbing fit. Instead, I feel a slight murmur of pain in my heart, a thin, whispery echo of a distant wound. It is then replaced by a warm, cathartic feeling like the one you get when you walk in the door on Thanksgiving morning. You're home.

I smile and say, "You're right. I don't have a baby in my belly anymore." And I know then that I've come a long way toward healing.

Laura isn't allowed to donate blood for Sarah because she's pregnant, so since I'm the same blood type, I volunteer to take her place. It isn't likely Sarah will even need it, but I feel better knowing if she does, it's coming from me.

You're supposed to wait six weeks after having a miscarriage to donate blood, but I figure I can just lie and they'll never know. My acupuncturist is not happy with that plan. She says it's a very bad idea, given I'm already low on blood and I'll be trying to get pregnant again soon. I ignore her advice and schedule the donation anyway. It's the least I can do.

I force down red meat and vegetables for lunch and dinner three days in a row to make sure I'm not anemic. The last thing I want is to get all the way to Houston where the donation is required and have them tell me I'm not eligible. I even call a blood bank in Austin to plead my case and see if they'll run a test on me to check for anemia. A sweet woman tells me what to say when I arrive so that I can get the test without actually giving blood. I'm thrilled when my drop of blood sinks to the bottom of the test tube, indicating I'm all clear.

***

Bright and early on a Saturday morning, my mother-in-law picks me up from the Houston airport, bringing me a delicious bag of donut holes to eat on our way to the donation center. I hold my breath when my drop of blood doesn't sink to the bottom this time, but luckily the follow-up centrifuge test approves me for donation.

My sweet mother-in-law donates too, just in case.

It takes four and half minutes for me to give blood. The blood bank volunteer marvels at my speed as if I'm some alien species. (After all the procedures I've been through trying to get pregnant, I feel like an alien, being poked and prodded by humans.) He nervously picks up my bandage as if I'm going to squirt blood all over the place, but I'm already clotted and ready for a Band-Aid. I'd warned him I usually filled the bag quickly, but he's acting like I've set a new record. While my mother-in-law finishes up her donation, the poor guy giving blood between the two of us turns a pale green. As we're leaving, the nurses are covering his neck and arms with ice packs. I feel terrible for him, but I am so glad I don't feel any worse than when I walked in an hour ago. I munch on some fresh, warm cookies from the donation center while we drive back to Austin to catch a UT baseball game.

**

A week later, Chris and I are back in Houston. It's the night before Sarah's surgery and the West Virginia shootings are all over the news. I have a nightmare that I'm in a vast courtyard full of inconspicuous people and I hear gunshots in the background. I find a bomb that's set to go off in 65 seconds. I scream for all of the people to run, urging everyone to flee to safety. Moments later, there's a massive explosion behind me.

I continue running and arrive at a pretty park where

everyone seems calm and unaware of the chaos behind me. I find three friends who are all very clearly pregnant. One of them says, "Congratulations—I heard the great news!" I reply, "Thank you. Unfortunately, I miscarried." But then I point over my shoulder and say, "But I just saved all of those other people."

I guess part of me must feel guilty that I couldn't save Squirt. The next day I buy a red helium balloon, say a litte prayer for Squirt, and then let it go, watching it until it disappears into the clouds.

***

The day of Sarah's surgery is stressful, though I can in no way imagine what it's like for my sister knowing that Sarah's heart will be stopped and cut open. I hope I never have to experience anything like it as a mother.

Laura is sobbing and I hug her tight. I want to tell her it will all be okay. Please God, let it all be okay. Then I look up to heaven and remind him he owes me one.

SWEET SARAH

The heart surgery seems harder this time because Sarah understands exactly what is going on. I hate hospitals, maybe because my sister, Lorie, once screamed at me, telling me to leave and never return, when she was in the hospital with cancer. I've never liked them since; never wanted to return. In her defense, she doesn't remember it. She was heavily drugged. I'm not blaming her. I just don't like them and I doubt that will ever change.

The last time I was at this hospital, Sarah was just a baby and I watched as the nurses took her from the arms of her parents to begin the first surgery. It's an image I can't get out of my head. It didn't really help my thing with hospitals either. I looked in her parents' eyes and saw exactly what I expected to see. They were terrified, and in turn that terrified me.

I'm told that Sarah is out of surgery and it's my turn to go back and see her. Two are allowed in the room at a time, but only one can go back at a time. So we've arranged shifts—I'll go back in someone's place and then the other person there will leave and Michelle will go back. I try to get out of it, murmuring some excuse, but I'm told quite firmly that it is my turn.

"She is sleeping anyway," Laura says.

So I head back through the bleach white hallways to Sarah's ICU room. On the way, I stop at a sink in the hallway and wash my hands multiple times. I take long strides and deep breaths trying to steel myself for what I will see. They needed the blood Michelle donated, which somehow makes me think the surgery was worse than they expected. And after all, this is open-heart surgery and she's just a child.

As I enter the room I see Sarah, her face is hers but she has tubes coming from her chest, machines flashing and beeping and fresh bandages covering her entire chest. Michelle's mom is there; she asks me if I've washed my hands. I nod; some things will never change.

She leaves to go and get Michelle—the idea is we'd get to see Sarah together. I still don't know why I got to go before her.

I look at Sarah and she seems so tiny with so many machines beeping and blinking hovering over her, a full maze of wires and tubes running to her chest, arms and nose. It looks like some sort of mechanical squid is emerging from her chest. I see a little girl boldly facing something that even scares me.

Sarah's eyes flicker open. Oh crap! So much for her being asleep. There is no panic in her, just a calm softness. This is exactly what I wanted to avoid. I shouldn't be the one here when she wakes up. I feel like I am violating some rule, and to be honest I'm afraid that she'll be upset. But she's not; somehow she's just fine with it.

I ask her how she is feeling. She softly says, "Fine."

A male nurse sees her awake and comes over. He checks her vitals and asks her how she's feeling. She doesn't answer until he puts her chart back and heads back to the nurse's station.

"Excuse me, Mister, I'm thirsty," she says in a fragile voice. I have a feeling that she can't get out the words, "Can I have some water please?" or they would follow.

The nurse brings her over a cup of ice. He tells her to suck on some of the ice chips, but after a few seconds of this Sarah pleads for a drink.

Where is Michelle? It seems like it's been too long since her mom went to find her.

I keep talking to Sarah. I ask her if I can hold her hand. She reaches out and I hold it gently. She's warm.

Finally the nurse relents; he brings her a small cup of ice water with a straw.

"Okay I'm going to give you some water, but just a little bit." He holds the straw up to her lips. As soon as the straw hits her lips I can see her gulp. Watching her drink makes me thirsty.

The water drains quickly from the cup. The nurse is now trying to pull the straw away but Sarah's lips are clinging to it, sucking as much liquid out as she can. He finally separates the straw from her and she relaxes. She lays back and I smile as big a smile as I can. I feel that the crisis is over. But she's very quiet and still.

Then it looks like she is trying to say something.

"How are you feeling?" I ask.

Then Sarah throws up.

Now I know why she was only supposed to drink a little bit. Throwing up sets off a bunch of things at the same time. First the nurse runs over, putting towels in her lap to catch anything else that comes out. He says something about protecting the bandages. So I hold one of the towels under her chin.

Sarah begins to cry and says, "Mister—I'm sorry I made a mess."

Only Sarah could think to apologize in this situation.

Michelle walks into the room and I see her expression turn from smiling to concern.

I smile. What else can I do?

I quickly explain to her what happened and volunteer to go get Laura. As I walk through the hallway I make a decision. I'm not going to tell Laura anything about Sarah being upset or her throwing up. I want her to be happy when she walks into Sarah's room, not frantic.

This ends up being a good decision, or so I'm told.

The surgery was a success, and a few weeks later Sarah is fully recovered, running around pell-mell like a four-year-old should.

LESSON 40: THANK GOD (OR YOUR DEITY OF CHOICE) FOR HAPPY ENDINGS.

THE WAITING GAME BEGINS AGAIN

Although we only need to wait a month before trying again, my acupuncturist recommends three months of treatment first. The words that sway me the most are, "Don't you want to make sure that if a miscarriage is avoidable next time, you've done all you can?" What possible answer is there to that but yes?

The acupuncture clinic's success rate is 100% for those who undergo treatments for three months versus a 40% miscarriage rate for those who have acupuncture treatments for less than three months. I'd only gone for a month before IVF. So, with a sigh and a lot of arm twisting (mostly my left arm twisting my right), I agree.

My acupuncturist's theory about my miscarriage is that my temperatures after ovulation aren't high enough (over 98 degrees) to support the production of hormones necessary to maintain a pregnancy. Meanwhile, my fertility doctor and gynecologist said there was a 99% chance the embryo just had a genetic defect. Was it a genetic fluke or is it something wrong with me? Who am I to believe?

I start tracking my basil body temperature every

morning (well, not every morning, because it takes me some time to automatically remember to take my temperature before I roll out of bed).

Part of me hopes the acupuncturist is right—at least there would be some kind of explanation for why I haven't been able to get pregnant and stay pregnant. And this is a problem that's actually fixable. But it turns out my temperatures are just fine. I'm tempted to renege on the three-month idea, but they talk me back into it, noting the other positives—like the fact that my cycle is longer for the first time in years.

Speaking of a longer cycle, maybe I'm pregnant. It's been 28 days since my last period, four days longer than usual. We weren't supposed to be trying to get pregnant, but Chris conveniently forgot the plan when we were fooling around a few days before I ovulated. The acupuncturist feels my pulse and says, "Are you sure you aren't pregnant?" I shrug and my heart beats a little faster at the thought. Now that my body has been pregnant once, maybe I've broken the spell. Can I really avoid future fertility treatments? The mere thought has me giddy.

I go home, walk straight into the bathroom, pull out my stash of pregnancy tests (I have at least ten sticks ready to go) and unwrap the white foil with zeal. Five minutes later, I've crashed back to reality. Will one of these sticks ever cooperate?

Well, at least I had a long cycle...

A FAMILY ADDITION

It's the heart of summer and we're crowded into a hospital room waiting for Laura to deliver Baby Boy Moorman. Although her due date isn't until next week, she came in to the hospital last night because she thought her water had broken. That wasn't the case, but when one of the tests showed a low amount of fluid in the pregnancy sac, they admitted her.

So we got the call this morning at 8:00 a.m. that the baby was coming early. Everyone but her husband, Lew, missed the worst of it, since Laura had been in major pain before the epidural.

My job is to take videos once the baby is born. Until then, I pass the time catching up on work.

Three hours of pushing later, John Wood Moorman is born. My mom was gushing with tears through the process watching Laura's face turn apple red. She was worried that my sister was having to push so hard (even though Laura swore she couldn't feel a thing). Halfway through the process, my mom says, "Michelle, I hope it won't be so hard for you." I have to remind her that I can't have natural childbirth anyway; pushing isn't going to be my problem.

For those keeping score, it's Laura—3, Michelle—0. If Squirt was still alive, I'd be six months pregnant now and John would have a cousin his age to play with.

SOMETHING IS DEFINITELY MISSING

We drive to San Antonio for the third time to see the birth of a Moorman child. I'm not upset that Laura and Lew are having a child before us, for the third time. I'm not upset that now we can't have the first boy in the family. I'm not upset that they are finished having kids before we have one.

Some people will be insensitive about this whole process. And insensitive to the fact that they can have children without going through drastic measures.

You are going to wonder if people think you don't deserve kids. You'll wonder if your friends who believe in God think that God doesn't want you to have kids. You'll wonder if people want you to be successful. Because some people truly can't be happy for others' success and that may include having children.

But as I write this, I am happy for anyone who can have a child. Even though we haven't and even if we can't. I've accepted that this is a possibility. I am still rooting for you, for anyone. Because I believe children are truly miracles. And I'll always root for miracles.

There is only one thing that upsets me. We still DON'T KNOW ANYTHING. Something is wrong with this process. Something has to be wrong with us and we still don't know what it is.

I watch Michelle holding John. She's happy for her sister, but there is that glint in her eye. A look you have to know someone deeply to be able to see. It's the "something's definitely missing" look. This isn't new. I've seen it for a while.

My job is to make Michelle happy, so I need to devise a plan. What that plan is, I have no idea. But I'm up for the challenge. She's worth it.

I won't let chance dictate the happiness of the people around me. I believe you make what you want of this world. And if this is my challenge, then I accept it fully.

Now I just have to figure out what to do if the IF happens.

LESSON 41: I NEED A PLAN.

THE CIRCUS—ACT II

It's month five post-miscarriage and our second month of "officially trying" to get pregnant with just acupuncture alone. My cycles are a little longer, my temperatures are looking great and I'm in good spirits.

Chris and I have just watched a DVD that highlights the key points from *The Secret*. If you aren't familiar with this self-help book, the key concept is that one's positive thoughts are powerful magnets that attract wealth, health and happiness through the laws of attraction. The video is a bit repetitive, but in general, it left me feeling more positive.

Then as usual on this roller coaster journey of infertility, just when things seem to be going well, the ground beneath my feet crumbles. Not only am I not pregnant, but my cycle is a very short 21 days.

That's the resounding end of this waiting game. It's time to start IVF again. Round two. I start birth control pills, get my schedule, and we're on our way. I'm excited for a couple of days, but of course this is the easy part.

Then I start reading the book, *Is Your Body Baby Friendly?*, which focuses on immunological disorders causing fertility issues. For the first time, I'm reading possible biological reasons that would completely explain why we haven't gotten pregnant and even why I miscarried after our first IVF try.

At an appointment with one of the IVF nurses for some paperwork and a short refresher course, we finally find out more about my first miscarriage. Remember that blighted ovum I mentioned earlier? I remember seeing so little on the ultrasound screen and after some research, I have a feeling the embryo never developed.

I ask the IVF nurse if this is a possibility and she leaves to grab my chart.

She returns and confirms my suspicion—we see a sonogram picture of an empty sac. It was a blighted ovum—cells formed the pregnancy sac, but not the embryo itself.

This deflates me.

It might not be reality, but it seems like "less progress" to me than if the baby had just stopped growing because it didn't have some random gene it needed to develop further.

But life moves on and we've gotta do what we've gotta do. And somehow I'm okay with all of this. Somehow I know I'll be okay. Maybe I've just dropped so low, or maybe it's that I can finally accept whatever happens, happens.

I'll live, I'll survive and I'll always have Chris.

So the circus act begins all over again.

STILL HEALING

Every time I see a child, I am reminded of how close we were. Or at least how close it seemed to me. Normally, I would appreciate this reflection time, but I can't now. I remember Squirt and I remember the pain. We wait several months for Michelle's body to heal. And now we are back at the doctor's office.

Michelle asks the doctor, "What would you suggest?"

"We try again," he says without hesitation.

"What could it have been?" Michelle pushes.

"Most miscarriages are a result of genetic disorders."

"I've been reading about problems with the woman's immune system attacking the embryo."

"It happens, but it is unlikely." He seems very certain about this. But as usual, he is uber patient with us.

"Do you think Chris and I should get tested for genetic abnormalities? Could that have been the issue?" Michelle is still prodding for an answer.

"I don't think that's the problem. But if you want to test for something, just let me know."

This is why he is our doctor. He helps us through the process. He gives us advice when we ask for it. But then he lets us make the final decision.

Dr. Vaughn agrees to order a few tests. Maybe we'll find a reason for our infertility—something that a half of one aspirin can help to solve.

Michelle finds out the <u>genetic testing</u> is covered by our insurance, so we both go in to give our blood. The results come back showing no genetic disorders. Her immune system check doesn't reveal any issues either.

No new answers. We're helplessly running out of items on the list. But something has changed. I realize Michelle's not asking as many questions as before. She's accepted it.

And suddenly, as if a switch in my head was triggered, I'm not the person who accepts what happens. I want a choice. I want freedom. I want to believe we have control no matter how unrealistic this really is. I'm frustrated and furious. It can't end like this. I want to pursue it as long as it takes, even if that isn't a rational approach.

All that is left to do is try in vitro again and hope that Michelle gets pregnant. And more importantly, stays pregnant.

LESSON 42: THE MILLER CURSE CONTINUES.

PART V

WORTH THE WAIT

IVF #2

We go through the entire IVF regiment again and this time it gives off a "been there, done that" kind of feeling. Probably because we know what to expect.

My body is reacting to the fertility medications more strongly this time—I'm extremely irritable and moody. I wouldn't want me for a wife right now. This is the kind way of saying I'm being a raging bitch.

We have some friends who've recently started down the infertility path who know they have a genetic disorder that might prevent them from conceiving. When I find out that genetic tests are almost completely covered by our insurance (we'd only be responsible for a $20 co-pay), I beg Dr. Vaughn to order the blood test for the two of us. Why not? Chris' aunt had Down syndrome.

And we've had almost every other test and still have no idea why we don't have a baby in our arms yet.

The doctor would turn out to be right, that this wasn't our issue, but I was happy to have one less thing to worry about. There are literally no other checkmarks to tick off that I can think of. We are the epitome of <u>unexplained infertility</u>.

At my first stimulation sonogram, there is a 45ish med student or sonogram student who joins Dr. Vaughn. I can tell right away that he doesn't have much experience. First, he has to peek under the paper drape and poke around to get the "fairy godmother wand" in the right spot. I feel like a Cadillac getting an oil change. Then, he doesn't move it around in order to see all the follicles like Dr. Vaughn does. Basically, anything he can see with the first angle is all he calls out, so according to him, I only have six follicles.

SIX?!

We've always had at least 10 follicles and this time my dose is significantly increased. I'm on the brink of crying or screaming, or both.

Dr. Vaughn points out one follicle that the student missed. I'm praying that there are really more and he just doesn't want to show the student up.

I ask the doctor if he is concerned with the lack of production and he replies, "No, but we'll increase your dose to 300 the next three nights and see what happens."

More shots. More sonograms. More follicles.

At our final sonogram check, my estradiol is pretty high (2,900), but we have 16 follicles with the lead follicle at 20mm and we are ready for the trigger shot.

It's time for egg retrieval again and sadly Sunny isn't working today. But we have a nice nurse who calls me honey and makes sure I have plenty of warm blankets. My anesthesiologist rocks, putting me under within a minute of walking in the surgical room before my feet are placed in the stirrups or my hands are splayed out to the side. It feels like a more humane process this time. It also feels at least 15 degrees warmer than last time, so I'm not shaking uncontrollably. This place was like a stay at a beach resort compared to last time. Good vibes.

When I get home, I flip through the mail and find a sweet card from my sister. There's a $5,000 check and a brief note that the money is just in case we want to do the genetic testing this time. I don't plan to cash it (we're planning to hold off on genetic testing until the next IVF cycle if there is a next one) but it is incredibly thoughtful of her.

EVERYTHING JUST FEELS RIGHT

After my performance I head back to the sterile room to wait for Michelle. They wheel Michelle in and she is all smiles. That happy, slightly drunk girl you wish you could take home smile. She's drugged all right.

She is not only happy but she's already asked me twice if Dr. Vaughn has come in with the report. He hasn't and I've answered both times. She's also just told me for the third time that we have a masseuse coming over tomorrow. I've already told her twice that she said it before.

So I just smile and say, "That is great news. I am very excited about it." She knows my voice and realizes she's been repeating herself. She laughs at herself and sighs a happy sigh.

A knock at the door. What do they think we could be doing? It's not as if we could possibly be having sex right now.

Dr. Vaughn enters, smiling, but I can't read anything else from him face.

"Everything went great and we retrieved 16 eggs."

Wow, I'm impressed. I just gave millions of sperm but they don't mean anything without one good egg and we have sixteen to choose from—we hope. They'll call us in 24 hours with the fertility report. I'm optimistic about this. I have to be. But, still, everything just feels right.

Tonight we start the progesterone shots again. Determined to make it through as many shots as we need to, Michelle collects more advice—massaging the area, sitting on a heating pad before and after and, logically, staying as far away as possible from that big nerve that runs down your back and leg. The goal—no more debilitating butt pain.

The next day, we get even better news, pushing me to be even more optimistic. We have 15 eggs that fertilized. We only need one good one.

THE SURPRISE EMBRYO

No call from the fertility clinic yet, so I take a trip to our acupuncture clinic bright and early this morning "just in case" we are told that our day 3 transfer appointment is on. As I'm walking out of the clinic, I hear from the fertility nurse that we're rescheduled for Friday. Oh well—an extra acupuncture appointment certainly can't hurt. Maybe this means my uterus will be ultra-relaxed and elastic like a rubber band.

Our embryos are higher in number and quality this time around. I wonder if this is due to (a) chance, (b) the fact that the lab had only been open for a few days before our first in vitro try (Chris still puts his money on this one), (c) the consistent acupuncture appointments Chris and I have both had over the past seven months or (d) some combination of the above.

Whatever the reason, I'm ecstatic.

Here is our run-down:

· 1 Embryo that is 8-cell, Grade 1, Compacting
· 1 12-cell, 1 9-cell, 5 8-cell, 1 7-cell and 1 6-cell Grade 1, Not Compacting
· 1 9-cell, 1 8-cell and 1 7-cell Grade 2, Compacting
· 1 9-cell, Grade 3, Compacting
· 1 9-cell and 1 6-cell Grade 3, Not Compacting

Hey wait. That's 16 embryos. We were told only 15 eggs had fertilized.

#16—the one that they didn't think fertilized on day 1—is the one with the most cells—the 12-cell/ Grade 1. Chris thinks that will end up being the winner—he was a late bloomer (he was only 5 feet tall in high school and ended up at 6'2") and so expects that his child might be the same.

When Chris comes home from work that night, he walks in the door and says, "You know what the first thing I'm going to say to number 16 is?"

"Who's number 16?" I ask baffled, thinking he's

talking about some sports player.

He rolls his eyes and explains, "Our 16th embryo. I'd say, you had me at 12 cells."

I laugh out loud.

I was a little teary when the IVF nurse told me that even #16, the one embryo they didn't think had fertilized the first day, had made it. Life always finds a way, right? I just hope "life finds a way" inside me instead of just in the Petri dish.

I'm very curious if they track each embryo individually so we'll know which ones looked the best on day 3 versus day 5. I think the answer is no, because my understanding is that there are several embryos in each Petri dish, but I'm definitely planning to ask the embryologist that question on Friday.

I was telling Chris on a walk a couple days ago that I think our luck is changing. I claimed, "We'll win the Austin Film Festival trailer competition, you'll have a great quarter at work, my marketing campaign will go really well and then we'll get pregnant." I would strike out on three of my four predictions.

PRACTICE MAKES PERFECT

Since we've started this process, we've had a few other friends who are in the same infertility boat.

Remember that friend with the cigar? He's since found out he has a genetic issue which means they have to go straight to in vitro. They've asked him to come in and make a "donation" and he doesn't understand the need for this.

I explain, "It's a practice run. They want to make sure you can perform when it counts. Imagine you get there, your wife is all ready and you can't finish."

He's quiet, but skeptical. I can tell he doesn't believe me.

I try describing the awkwardness of the whole place. "It's a room with a chair, and a thin wall. You put the specimen into a drawer like a bank teller and on the other side is a lab technician waiting for you to finish."

I can tell he is not buying it, but he probably won't have any trouble. I just wanted him to be prepared.

A week later, I'm at my desk when he calls. I know it's his practice day, so I answer the phone.

"It was a disaster. I had to leave. I couldn't do it."

We meet for lunch and he tells me he was too

embarrassed to go back in and tell them he couldn't do it so he called them from the car. By the end of lunch we're both laughing hysterically. There is something genuinely funny about making fun of ourselves. I'm happy to say a few days later—when it counted—he had no problems at all.

LESSON 43: AS LONG AS YOU CAN LAUGH AT YOURSELF, YOU WILL NEVER CEASE TO BE AMUSED.

HOLDING MY BREATH

Everything seems to go well the day of the transfer. I even make it through the hour wait afterwards before getting up to pee. The best two embryos are much closer in size and quality than the first IVF round. They turn out to be the 12-cell and 9-cell embryos from day 3—the most advanced embryos from the original report. That means "#16" is one of them! And they came from the same Petri dish, so if we end up having twins, they'll have been together since the very beginning. Was it written in the stars?

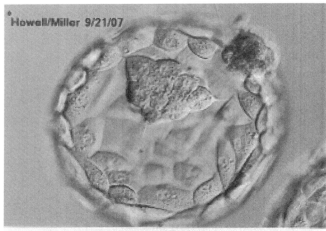

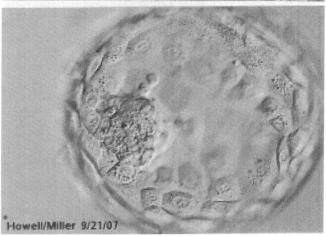

Our Two Embryos from IVF #2

When Chris mentions to our doctor how excited he is about #16, our late bloomer, we get a different version of the events than we'd thought had occurred. Dr. Vaughn smiles and says, "Actually, that embryo had probably already fertilized. We look for certain signs that an embryo has fertilized and sometimes we think one hasn't fertilized because it has already passed that point. So if your #16 was a 12-cell embryo, it was ahead of the game. That's why we keep on watching all of them—just in case."

Chris doesn't remember the conversation going this way. He even blocks out that the conversation was with Dr. Vaughn. And most days, he still likes his version of the story—the slow starter—better. But he did note that if Dr. Vaughn is right, that just means Baby Girl or Baby Boy Miller is more like me. He thinks of me as an overachiever because I went to college when I was 16 and graduated when I was 19. So, in either case, #16 takes after one of us in a big way.

We have ten days to go until the pregnancy test. I'm going batty with anticipation but I get a sign that makes me smile and think positively. The man who picks up our football tickets for the weekend bought them so he could take his two-year-old twins to their first football game. We'll have to watch it on TV because I'm constrained to puttering around the house for 24 hours after the transfer. I am tempted to ask him how they ended up with twins, but since I've only just met him, I figure that's as inappropriate as someone asking me if I'm ovulating.

Now all we can do is hope, pray and wait. In everyday life, ten days seems to pass before I've blinked, but I'm only on day 4 and it feels like it could have been a month already. A snail travels faster than this. It feels like I'm holding my breath.

LIFE FINDS A WAY

Dr. Vaughn removed 16 eggs. The next day, we were told 15 of them fertilized. But a few days later, we're told that there are, in fact, 16 embryos.

Did I mention that I was five feet one inch as a high school freshman? Did I mention that I took a lot longer than my father wanted to finish college? Did I mention I'm a procrastinator? That I save the best for last? I waited until halfway through college to start studying and get As. Only the fruit of my loins could follow in my footsteps.

And so here is the sixteenth embryo, showing up late to the show but on the brink of a grand performance. This, I am dead certain, is my kid. Anyone who can befuddle the doctors into thinking there is no chance and then, BAM, there is more than a chance—there is LIFE. I'll call it Number 16. That's the nickname. It's not just that it was late. It's also that the fertilization looked impossible. Like us—having a kid looked impossible.

When we arrive on the transfer day, I hope that they

tell us they are putting in Number 16. This one is going to be strong. He or she will love to prove people wrong. What more could I ask for?

The doctor is explaining something about how Number 16 was probably fertilized early and they just could not see the sperm entering the egg. I stare him down, my face dripping with a deadpan expression. What the hell does he know? Absolutely nothing. I like my version better.

But I guess even if Number 16 was the early one, then it's Michelle's doppelganger. She skipped a couple grades. She went to college early. She graduated early.

So either way, it's our child.

But I still think the doctor is wrong. After all, he told me that my sperm only live for two to three days and I still see some of them swimming around in the Petri dish.

"I thought that sperm only lived for three days. Hasn't it been five?" I chide our doctor.

Dr. Vaughn turns to Michelle and says, "He'll be bragging about this for weeks."

Then he tells us they are indeed putting in Number 16. It feels lucky.

Come on Number 16—find a way.

LESSON 44: NOTHING IS IMPOSSIBLE.

FINALLY RIGHT ABOUT SOMETHING

It's finally day 10 and if I could hold my breath between the time I give blood in the morning and the time we hear the results, I probably would. Actually, if I could just sleep peacefully for the six hours in between, that sounds like an even better plan.

Chris takes the afternoon off so we can call in together.

And then we hear the news.

Out of my four predictions, the only one I was right about was the most important one. I am pregnant again. And this time my hCG level is a stronger 175. I wonder if that means twins? All I care about is that I can carry at least one healthy baby to term.

THERE IS NO GIRL FROM FLORIDA

With my first pregnancy, I had only distant, meandering thoughts about the possibility of a miscarriage. I figured surely we would catch a break after what we'd gone through to get pregnant in the first place. Now that I've been through one, it preys on my mind.

The blood tests have all been going well so far—the hCG numbers are going up like they should and my progesterone levels are strong (and luckily the shots haven't been much of an issue thanks to Nurse Chris). But I find myself losing sleep the night before each test and then tensing up my shoulders right before hearing the results. It's that little fear that chews on the back of my brain.

One difference is that I feel more pregnant this time. I have waves of nausea throughout the day. My breasts are sore and ballooning up like a moon bounce. I'm in week 6 before I know it. This is the time where things went south in IVF #1, and I catch myself holding my breath.

My hCG number is within normal range, but it didn't quite double, so I'm on the Internet furiously checking to see what exactly that could mean. My pro-gesterone level is off-the-charts high for how early I am in my pregnancy, even though the doctor cut my dose in half, and there doesn't seem to be a good explanation why. Now we have to wait another seven days for my next hCG test and two weeks for the heartbeat sono-gram. I mention my fears to Mandy, one of the acu-puncturists (the best one with the needles) and she tells me the following story:

"I'd just moved from California to Austin and I was looking for an apartment downtown. At the time, they were really hard to find in that location. Anything that went on the market rented within an hour or two. I found this great place with hardwood floors, beauti-ful doorway arches and crystal door handles. But the woman told me there was a girl from Florida ahead of me. I went home disappointed.

I was in the shower later that night and I told myself, 'There is no girl from Florida,' over and over again. I felt better. I felt positive. And three days later, I called the woman back and she let me know the apartment was mine if I wanted it. The girl from Florida hadn't called her back. That positive energy made my wish come true."

Wish it, repeat it and it just might come true. This baby is healthy and strong. This baby is healthy and strong.

Sometimes this acupuncture clinic feels like a shrink's office, which I might need even more than help on my Qi. A little crazy from the hormones and the anxiety and the waiting, I can use every last drop of advice to keep me sane.

***

It's my niece, Sarah's, birthday and we're in San Antonio for a family dinner to celebrate. This time with IVF, I included only our parents and my sister in my email updates because we figured it was better to keep the group small until we passed the three-month mark. So while Chris and my sister knew I was pregnant, nobody else at the table did.

We have a room all to ourselves and there are about 20 of us stretched out down a long table. Everyone is chatting and gossiping and munching on appetizers. I'm struggling to find something that sounds good on the menu when shy Sarah says, "Michelle, are you pregnant?"

The boisterous conversations along the table suddenly halt. The room is silent.

Did my sister put her up to this? I reply with my voice cracking and nervous, "Why do you ask?"

And then, in her usual way of making me melt into a puddle of loving goo, she says, "Because we've been praying for you every night."

So I can't help but look into her sparkling blue eyes and say, "Well, I could be."

As a result of my response, the room explodes into a maelstrom of questions, so I give them the run-down of our latest IVF adventure.

Nancy, my sister's sweet mother-in-law, asks, "How are you feeling?"

I reply frankly, "Terrible!"

Knowing that usually means the pregnancy is in full swing, she says, "Oh good!"

I return to my menu to try to find something that sounds like it might stay down. Baked potato it is.

NUMBER 16'S FIRST BIG BREAKFAST

Michelle feels like shit, which is great. I'll bet this is the only time I will be able to say that.

She's been going in for tests every couple of days. The alarm goes off and I know she's getting up for another test.

"Good luck!" I say as she heads out the door.

We're approaching the six-week mark, which is when we discovered the miscarriage last time.

I hear the front door close. I roll out of bed. I can't sleep.

I'm going to make Michelle breakfast. Manual labor is one sure way I can deal with stress. Exercise, even when it's just whipping up waffles, is my escape from living in my thoughts.

An hour later, Michelle comes back through the door.

"Did you do good?" I yell to her.

Michelle comes into the kitchen smirking.

"I've made you and Number 16 breakfast."

"I can see that."

I went crazy with the food. Neither of us could polish off the smorgasbord even if we ate leftovers for a week.

"But you still think you're pregnant?" I can tell she was thinking about it too.

"Yes. I am still very nauseous. That went away last time."

"It'll be fine this time. After all, it's Number 16."

LESSON 45: DISTRACT. DISTRACT. DISTRACT.

I LIKE THIS ONE MUCH BETTER

The Internet is my favorite tool because it lets me shop, catch up with friends and check on the status of my fetus all in one. It's also dangerous for people like me. These days, the slightest twinge or tweak or pain, my hypochondriac irrationality takes me to the net to look up possible problems.

It's a week before our heartbeat sonogram is scheduled and my left side has been aching for 24 hours. I know from research on my last miscarriage that this can be a side effect of an ectopic pregnancy, but that is supposed to be a sharp pain versus the dull pain I have now. Since it's a Sunday, my only choice is to page the IVF nurse.

When I explain what I'm feeling, she suggests calling Dr. Vaughn, but asks me to wait an hour or two until he's out of church. When I reach him, he asks several probing questions. I'm certain he is developing a highly complicated diagnosis. He then tells me it's most likely just constipation. I guess my paranoia is as bloated as my stomach.

"But if you're worried about it, come on in for a sonogram tomorrow and we'll get you checked out," he says kindly.

***

In the morning, I call for a sonogram appointment and they squeeze me in that afternoon. I am excited and energized and nervous and scared. But I can't wait to see the baby and possibly hear the heartbeat.

Our friends Jennifer and David had a miscarriage with their first pregnancy and they didn't find out until the day they went in for their first sonogram, when they saw their baby on the screen with no heartbeat.

When she got pregnant five months later and it was time for a sonogram, upon seeing the heartbeat David replied, "I like this one much better!" I'm not sure if he was talking about the baby or the sonogram or both, but I hope to have that same feeling a few hours from now.

It is still early for a heartbeat—we're right at that border—so no heartbeat won't necessarily mean bad news. But wouldn't it be heavenly to see and hear the heartbeat now so I don't have to spend the next week wondering.

Chris and I hold hands.

The doctor turns the screen our way. We lean in with rapt attention and see what looks like a fetus the size of a lima bean on the screen. And there, in the center of the lima bean's tiny chest is a pulsing dot—a heart. Mine swells with joy.

We hear the swoosh, swoosh, swoosh, swoosh of the quick heartbeat.

There's our #16.

Chris asks if there's any chance that we just can't see the other embryo and the doctor says it's very unlikely. He puts the odds at less than 1%. While there were some positives to having twins, I'm thrilled to be able to give this little one my undivided attention for a while.

16 WEEKS IN

It's exactly 16 weeks into the pregnancy today. If we are lucky, we will find out if Number 16 is a girl or a boy. We are at a specialist's office—giant flat screen TVs adorn the eggshell white walls—to check out Number 16's development and test for any abnormalities.

The nurse comes in and spreads the familiar blue jelly on Michelle's stomach. She straps on a heartbeat monitor and we can hear Number 16's quick-beating heart. What sounds very fast is absolutely normal—a normal fetal heart rate is 110-160 beats per minute, depending on the gestational age. And after a few minutes, it sounds rhythmic and quite soothing.

She measures each body part and then compares it on a chart. Arms. Legs. Head.

Number 16 is exactly average—in the fiftieth percentile. And there are no signs of any genetic disorders.

Michelle and I look at each other. I peer into her eyes and can see all the pain and struggle dissolve. This moment is our catharsis. In this moment, we have our first bit of peace.

And then the nurse clicks a button and snaps a frame of Number 16's legs.

"It's a girl."

I see the profile of her face. She has a tiny nose and she's beautiful.

My eyes fill with tears. There's my girl. My girl. That has such a different meaning now. I've met magical Number 16. And she is doing well.

Average is perfect. She is perfect. This moment is perfect. I just want her to grow healthy and strong. And get here soon. I can't wait to meet you Sydney.

LESSON 46: SOMETIMES GOOD THINGS REALLY DO COME TO THOSE WHO WAIT.

THE COUNTDOWN BEGINS

I'm sure we could write an entire book about the pregnancy, but mine is a cakewalk compared to the process of getting pregnant.

Dr. Binford, my new OB, takes good care of me.

The first trimester flies by.

My nausea subsides at 14 weeks.

The second trimester is relatively painless. That nagging fear of another miscarriage packs up her bags and quietly exits my mind. People who don't know me start to notice my belly. I read books about babies and breastfeeding and parenting.

The weight and size of Sydney finally makes it difficult to sleep or walk or sometimes even to breathe. My back aches. My legs and feet swell up like a blowfish. My tummy grows larger and larger, visible signs of our journey to pregnancy. I'm happily miserable. I rest as much as possible, which thankfully I can do since I work for myself.

We talk to Sydney every day. I rub my belly and tell her stories. I sing her lullabies every night in the bathtub. Sydney hiccups a lot.

Check up after check up goes well. They start out every month. Then every two weeks. Then every week.

With a month left to go, Sydney is still breech, and her head, arms and legs are all bunched up under my left ribcage. It feels like there's an alien taking a hammer to my ribs. I will be ecstatic to get her out of my body and into my arms.

APPROACHING THE END

Through the pregnancy I'm still cautious, but I've met

her, Number 16. I've bent over in the dark at night and whispered to her. I've told her she's smart, she's beautiful, she's happy, she's healthy and if she works hard, she can do anything.

There are no limits for her; all she has to do is get here. I'm nervous. Not about meeting her, but about knowing what to do when she gets here. But I know Michelle and I will figure it out, together.

LESSON 47: I HAVE NO IDEA HOW TO BE A FATHER, BUT IT STILL FEELS GREAT KNOWING I WILL BE ONE.

THE BIG DAY

June 1ˢᵗ, 2008—the big day is finally here. We're scheduled for a C-section this morning. All the trying. All the waiting. It's finally over.

I say a big prayer that everything goes well.

My parents and sister and Chris' parents are all here. I'm packed and ready. It's time to go to the hospital.

We check in. We wait. Dr. Binford walks in, squeezes my hand and asks if we're ready.

I'm ready. I've been ready for nearly four years.

The C-section itself was anxiety-ridden and uncomfortable and painful. But none of that matters, because an hour later, I'm holding our beautiful Sydney in my arms.

Her big gray eyes look into mine. Her tiny fingers latch onto my hand. Her wrinkled blue feet are bunched up, trying to return to their breech position. Her soft, warm skin presses against my face.

She is perfect in every way.

She was worth the wait.

SYDNEY ARRIVES

Tomorrow is the big day and we are picking Michelle's mom up from the airport. She gets in the car and mentions that tomorrow is Charlie's birthday. Charlie is Michelle's uncle, her father's brother. And something unpleasant surfaces.

I think, hold on, didn't Michelle's grandmother die giving birth to Charlie? Suddenly tomorrow doesn't seem like the right day to have a child. How on earth did no one think this through?

I blurt out, "Wait, tomorrow is Charlie's birthday?

And didn't Charlie's Mom die giving birth to him?"

"No Ladd's mother died giving birth to him. Charlie had a different mother."

I'm relieved. Just one coincidence I didn't need. Technology has come a long way but things happen and I don't want anything to happen to Michelle.

***

What's usually a lazy Sunday morning is anything but lazy. Today is June 1st—the day Sydney will come into this world.

Some of the mystery of the birth of our child may have slipped away. Unlike other couples, who will wait until labor ensues, we've known for the last three months that if Sydney doesn't come early, then she will come today. That's because through the trials of getting pregnant in the first place, Michelle's abdominal myomectomy has made a C-section a certainty.

Michelle's bag is packed and it feels like we are soldiers preparing for a mission. The Viacord kit is the only other thing we need to bring.

If you haven't thought about <u>cord blood banking</u>, I strongly recommend it. Basically the doctor collects the umbilical cord blood after the birth and then you ship it off to be stored. While it is expensive (~$2,000 plus $125/year in storage), it may save a family member's life one day. They are already doing amazing things with stem cells. Who knows what they'll be able to do by the time Sydney grows up and has her own children?

I don't know much about the process today except that we'll check in, the nurse will prepare Michelle for the C-section, she'll go back on her own to get her set up in the operating room and then they'll call me in to join her. I only know this much of the process because I insisted on asking. I still have no idea what to expect when it comes to the actual procedure.

Today is filled with anticipation and fear, like I am going on a trip to an uncertain destination. I do not underestimate the responsibility of having a child. My solace is that I will share this with Michelle, who I am certain will be a great mother.

As she waddles through our living room, tending to last minute details like making sure the cats have enough food and setting our AC a little higher, I realize that she might seem less nervous because any fear is overcome by her desire to get the giant, heavy basketball out of her uterus.

We pack up the car, say goodbye to her mother and sister who will bring a second car to the hospital, and head out in our last car ride as non-parents. It's quiet and we spend the time mainly holding hands.

We arrive on the second floor and there is no one at the check-in desk. I go around the corner to the nurse's station and one of them tells me they will call. A nurse starts prepping Michelle while I am supposed to fill out paperwork. Since I have never filled out any paperwork during this whole pregnancy, this is both new to me and very stressful. There are questions I have no idea how to answer.

I take the paperwork into Michelle's room, where she fills out the rest while we listen to the familiar heartbeat of our unborn child.

The nurse suddenly says, "Oh look there's another contraction."

Michelle and I stare at each other, shocked. Michelle shrugs her shoulders. She didn't feel anything this morning.

Dr. Binford comes in and begins checking Michelle.

"How has your weekend been?" I ask, trying to break the ice.

"Terrible," she replies.

What? Dr. Binford is always so cheerful, this is the last thing I expected to come out of her mouth. My mind races back to Michelle's grandmother dying giving birth to her father. That's what terrible means to me. But I don't dare ask anymore. I don't want to know.

"Okay. Are you ready to deliver this baby?" Dr. Binford asks.

And suddenly there is a huge relief. It's all really going to happen.

Then my stomach turns over. Now I am really nervous.

There is one last, brief moment where is it just me and Michelle, and then the craziness begins.

Two nurses come in followed by the anesthesiologist. I'm asking questions while they start an IV, but

I'm only barely listening to their answers. The anesthesiologist is explaining what will happen once he takes Michelle back.

I'm staring at Michelle, joyful and in the moment.

We kiss.

And now they are rolling her away.

They hand me some scrubs and I go to wash my hands. The procedure will take place in the operating room, so I need to be as sterile as I can be.

I'm waiting.

The nurse comes for me and asks, "Do you have your camera?"

"Wait, I can take pictures?" I figured there would be liability issues.

"Yes of course!"

I am an amateur; this is my first time.

Laura is running, literally, down the hall to get me her camera. This isn't helping my nerves. I can't imagine what else I've forgotten. But my train of thought it interrupted, I can hear Laura running down the hall back to me. I run to meet her.

She's smiles and says, "Good Luck!"

I follow the nurse into the operating room. I've been in operating rooms before, both as a patient and as an observer. But this one is a bit different; it reminds me of something alien. Michelle is strapped to the table, her arms tied. There are ten people in the room, clustered in different areas. I can hardly imagine what they will all be doing.

A green sheet is draped under Michelle's armpits as a curtain. It's supposed to hide what the doctor is doing. I'm too tall for it to hide anything. I contemplate telling them this when Michelle's doctor says, "Hi Chris. Have a seat and I will tell you when we are getting close."

Michelle tilts her head and she looks up at me with her big brown eyes. The anesthesiologist is talking to her; keeping her company. I'm still disoriented from what I just glimpsed on the other side of the sheet, but I try my best to put it out of my mind and smile down at Michelle.

The anesthesiologist reminds me I have a camera. I take a picture of Michelle. It won't be flattering, but it captures the moment. I realize I can take another cool photo, and I snap one of myself in my scrubs.

Michelle and I are listening to the doctor on the other side of the curtain. They're talking about pools and outdoor patios, but they are also working. I know they've already made the incision and I guess they must be moving her organs around inside.

"What do you do?" the anesthesiologist asks me.

"Huh? Oh, I'm a writer and I sell software." This is how I have decided I will answer people from now on. There is what I want to do and what I get paid for.

"Is everything going as planned?" I ask him tentatively.

He stands up and looks over the curtain. If I just looked that direction while I'm sitting down, I could see everything. So I don't. I stare at Michelle instead.

For more then three years we've waited to meet this little kid. And now the moment is nearly here.

"Everything is going great. You're doing great," he says.

"The truth is, you're not doing shit," I say to Michelle.

She smiles. "Tell me about it." She pushed her hands up in the air to show that they are strapped in.

I reach out and hold her hand.

"I love you anyway. I love you mostest." I smile.

I can hear scuffling and the anesthesiologist tells me I should stand up. I take a last glance at Michelle.

I peer over the curtain and I can see something white. Something being tugged. It's pink, no purple and white. And I see something brown and yellow too.

It's floppy.

And then the doctor tugs Sydney out. She flails, her mouth opens wide and I hear a SCREAM. It's pure fear. I've never heard anything quite like it.

I realize the brown and yellow I saw was my child having the shit and piss scared out of her. I feel horrible for her.

And then the nurse is beside me. She asks me, "Don't you want to take a picture?"

I must seem like an idiot. What the hell is she talking about? Why would I want to take this picture? This won't be flattering for my child—not now, not ever.

More screaming.

I squeeze Michelle's hand.

Michelle is sobbing. "Is everything okay?"

"You have a beautiful baby girl," Dr. Binford finally announces.

The nurse who asked me about the pictures is my bulldog. "Don't you want to come with your daughter?" she asks.

I do, but I don't want to leave Michelle's side. I have to go. Sydney is still crying.

I follow the nurse over to a small glass bin. There is a tiny baby lying in the middle. It's our baby. Sydney.

Her legs are purple and they are flopping, like they are made of rubber. They dangle out to her sides. It doesn't look normal. Nothing looks normal right now. But what could be normal at this moment?

In fact her head is not normal either. It's flat. She was pressing her head under Michelle's ribs for a long time and it shows. She looks like Predator, from the movie with Arnold Schwarzenegger.

The nurses are busy cleaning Sydney off. Putting on a diaper, wrapping her in clothing. She reminds me of a frog, or some kind of purple amphibian. I'm certain that something is wrong with her. This can't possibly be normal. So I ask, "Is she okay?"

"We'll need to give her a more thorough checkout, but she looks great."

She is still crying. We reached inside and pulled her out of a place where she was happy and warm and cozy and she hasn't gotten over it yet. Something else is nagging at me.

Then I watch as they cut her umbilical cord.

"Michelle, we forgot the Viacord!"

"Shit! Shit! Shit!" Michelle yells.

It's actually the anesthesiologist who comforts her. "Just think of it like it's ten years ago and there wasn't a cord blood option."

I feel awful. I'm already a horrible parent and it's been less than ten minutes.

"Do you want to see why she is crying?" asks the bulldog nurse.

"Yes." Anything to take my mind off of my mistake.

The nurse pushes Sydney's legs up, pinning her feet next to her ears. And then there is silence. It's the first moment of understanding. Her eyes are open and she is not crying, she just looks around.

"Her legs hurt her when they are pushed straight."

Sydney's been bunched up in a ball for so long, that her legs are used to being up by her head.

"But they'll be normal eventually, right?"

There is a new nurse now. She's the one cleaning and changing Sydney. "Most of the time. The worst case is that she'll need leg braces, but that is rare."

That won't do. I have a friend who had leg braces and because of that he hated the movie *Forest Gump*. She has to like *Forest Gump*.

Now we are wheeling Sydney over to Michelle. I can see what the doctor is working on behind the curtain. I wish I hadn't looked—again.

Michelle is still strapped in. She looks helpless. I know I am supposed to go with Sydney but I know I won't want to leave. Michelle wants to know everything, but what do I really know? I tell her they told me she is fine.

The nurse brings Sydney up to Michelle's face and all the questions stop. Silence. A moment between mother and daughter. I cry. I can't help it. Michelle and Sydney's faces touch.

The doctors and nurses give us a moment—just the three of us. This might be the whole reason they do what they do. To see this moment once a day must give your life a real charge.

I snap a few pictures to try and capture in pixels what my heart will never forget.

It's time for us to part. They need to finish sewing Michelle up and we need to take Sydney to the ICU to complete her check-up. I kiss Michelle and I tell her I love her and will see her soon.

We turn to go and I shout over my shoulder to her doctor. "Do a good job Doc!"

I only hope she smiles.

The nurse and I wheel Sydney in her glass tub down the hallway to the baby ICU. She's crying, but I can barely hear it.

At the end of the hall, I see Michelle's sister and mother. I really don't know what to say. We pause to give them a chance to see Sydney. I'm holding her little hand. Her hand is so small, so fragile. How can it hold anything, do anything? I realize at this moment she can't and that is why I am here. To protect her; provide for her.

They ask me all about her. I rattle off the stats I know, but my list is very short.

We're moving again and I ask the nurse if she has kids. She does. I ask her if it was weird to her. I apologize if I am being too honest or if this makes me a bad parent, but this whole thing seems bizarre.

"I really don't know this kid at all, but now she is mine. It's a whole lot to take in at one time."

She smiles at me; I can tell she has been here before.

I feel empathy for Sydney, from when she cried, when we yanked her out of that quiet comfortable world she was in. I wonder what she will like, what she will be like? Will she be like Michelle (strong-willed, determined, confident)? Like me (goofy, a dreamer, a procrastinator)? A little like both of us? How will her laugh sound? So much of a mystery; so much left to fill in.

The nurse begins to bathe her. I imagined a bathtub with soap and water, but this is no more than a few soft cloths with warm water and soap. Sydney is covered with what looks like chalk, like baby powder, white and soft. I wonder if this is where "baby powder" got its name.

Sydney is crying more loudly now and she begins to do something strange with her tongue—flicking it in and out of her mouth. It reminds me of what my aunt used to do. The problem is that my aunt had Down syndrome. And so I freak out all over again.

The world is already a huge challenge. She has a predator head and purple frog legs she may need braces for. Please tell me she doesn't have Down syndrome.

I ask the nurse about Sydney's tongue and she laughs. She tells me it's a good sign. It means she is hungry.

"It's called rooting. She is searching for food."

I put my hand in her palm and she closes her fingers around my thumb. For a moment she looks at me and stops crying.

I tell her what I have been waiting to say to her for ten months.

"Welcome to the world. I'm your father and I will love you always and forever. I am going to screw a lot of things up in your life, so I apologize for all of it now. I can only promise that I will try as hard as I can. You're smart, you're beautiful, we love you very much and you can do anything you want if you work hard. Don't ever give up."

I'll tell her that every day. Or at least every day until she is old enough to decide she won't listen to me anymore.

I hear a knock on the glass behind me. My parents have arrived and seeing them brings up my emotions. Especially seeing my dad. I am him years ago. And he is still happy.

I wonder for a minute if they are all smiling because they know we will now get paid back for how we acted as children.

Michelle's mom and sister are there too. They can hear Sydney crying, it's been ten minutes and I'm not doing very well. My dad urges me to comfort her. I am afraid. Sydney seems so fragile. I mention this to the nurse. She smiles. "You'll get used to it. You can hold her if you want."

I want Michelle to be the first to hold her, she was tied up and that's not fair. So I place my hand on her tummy to comfort her.

The nurse gets a call that Michelle is in the recovery room.

"We're going to go back to see Mom," I tell Sydney. I describe who Michelle is and where we are right now. I tell her about all of the people who are here to meet her. When we go into the hall, our family surrounds her.

Michelle sees Sydney and tears well up in her eyes. She's sitting up and her arms are finally untethered. The nurse hands Sydney to her. There is a glow. Something that can only be explained as love. And pure joy. She's been waiting for this for a long time.

I go over to Michelle and just lean close to them both. Sydney is breastfeeding; she looks up at both of us. And I know now why we went through all of this. It is for that one glimpse.

Our families give us some time alone.

Michelle and I kiss.

I apologize about the Viacord. I still can't believe it. The kit is in the car. We came so close. I just hope we never need it.

I mention to Michelle how weird this is to me. She asks me to explain, which I am not sure I can. The simplest way to put it is that we can't leave. We can't just go home. We'll have her forever if we are lucky. I don't want to leave because I already love her, but the responsibility is even bigger than I ever imagined. Better than I imagined.

Michelle smiles at my explanation.

"Even with her frog legs and predator head, I love her more than I imagined. And I have quite an imagination."

Sydney cries, reminding us she needs us.

LESSON 48: IT WAS ALL WORTH IT.

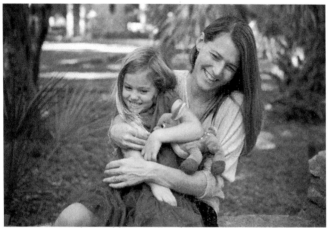

Sydney Addison Miller, Born June 1, 2008

EPILOGUE

(18 MONTHS LATER)

Sydney is now 18 months old. She is fun. She talks, A LOT. I'm busy entertaining her because Michelle doesn't feel well. She feels nauseous which is unusual, the last time was....

"No way," I say out loud to no one, but Sydney repeats it immediately. Note to self—watch what you say.

I head into the bedroom. Michelle is one step ahead of me, as usual. She is in the bathroom, peeing on a stick.

Sydney tags along behind me. She climbs up on the bed, and I climb on next to her. Michelle pops her head out of the bathroom.

"Not pregnant," she calls out. Oh well. We can hope, right? But we've only been trying for six months and if we can't do it on our own, we have three frozen embryos waiting for us. We've decided we'll cross that bridge when Sydney turns two.

Sydney and I begin to play one of our favorite games, 20 questions. It's where Sydney asks me twenty or more questions about everything she can think of, and each question is usually followed by another question which at some point gets to why.

"Daddy do birds poop?" She asks.

"Yes they do." I answer.

"But birds don't pee do they?" she asks. In case you're wondering, they don't.

"No they don't," I respond.

"Why?" she asks.

I'm about to answer when Michelle peeks her head out of the bathroom, smiling and holding the pee stick. She is pregnant. I wish she would learn to read those sticks.

I turn to Sydney. "Sydney we have some news for you."

Sydney's face gets very serious.

"Mommy is pregnant, and you're going to have a little brother or sister."

I pause waiting.

Sydney raises her hands in the air and shouts, "Yeah!"

I couldn't have said it better myself. I just wish I'd gotten it on video.

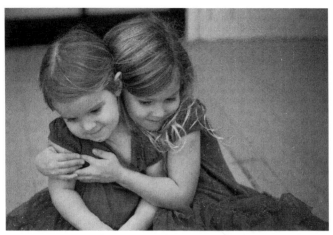

Sabrina Catherine Miller, Born September 8, 2010

(ANOTHER 20 MONTHS LATER)

Michelle's stomach has been acting up over the last two days and she is nauseous. She just stopped breastfeeding a week ago. Maybe it's the hormones? Her period is late, so she pulls out a pregnancy test just in case, all the while assuring me that she isn't pregnant.

I think back to a couple weeks ago. We'd fooled around without a condom when we thought we were in the safe, post-ovulation zone.

Five minutes later she has a stick in her hand, her eyes wider than I've ever seen them.

I announce, "Sydney, Sabrina, we have some news for you…"

A little sooner than we'd planned, but baby boy Luke was on his way, ready or not!

LESSON 49: LIFE DOESN'T ALWAYS GO THE WAY YOU EXPECT IT TO.

LESSON 50: CHERISH EVERY MOMENT.

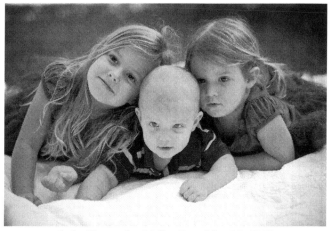

Luke Christopher Miller, Born May 22, 2012

APPENDIX A
DEFINITIONS & DESCRIPTIONS

Abdominal Myomectomy—Surgery through an open abdominal incision to access your uterus and remove one or more fibroids.

Acupuncture—Among the oldest healing practices in the world, acupuncture stimulates points on the body by pricking the skin or tissues with needles.

Basal Body Temperature (BBT)—The temperature of your body in the morning after awakening. The basal body temperature typically rises and falls due to changes in hormone levels during the menstrual cycle.

Blastocyst Transfer—A more recent advance in infertility treatment, which involves growing human embryos in the laboratory to a later "blastocyst" stage—typically day 5—before transferring them into the uterus following in vitro fertilization.

Blighted Ovum (egg)—A fertilized egg that implants itself in the uterus but does not develop properly.

Cesarean Section (C-Section)—A procedure in which a baby, rather than being born vaginally, is surgically removed from the uterus.

Clomiphene (Clomid)—The most widely prescribed fertility drug, it increases the production of gonadotropins to stimulate follicle growth and egg development.

Compacting Embryo—Once an embryo divides so many times, and the embryologist can no longer count the number of cells, it is considered a "compacting" embryo.

Cord Blood Banking—The storage of private or public umbilical cord blood for future use. Cord blood transplants are currently being used to treat diseases of the blood and immune systems.

Dilation and Curettage (D&C)—A procedure to dilate the cervix and scrape away the uterine lining, often performed after a first trimester miscarriage.

Ectopic Pregnancy—A pregnancy that occurs when a fertilized egg implants in a woman's body outside of the uterus.

Egg Retrieval—Use of a thin needle to remove eggs from the ovarian follicles for ICSI, IVF or other procedures.

Embryo Transfer—Placement of the fertilized egg (embryo) into the uterus using a catheter after IVF and other ART procedures.

Estradiol—An estrogen hormone secreted by the ovaries.

Endometriosis—The presence of endometrial tissue in abnormal locations such as the fallopian tubes, ovaries, and peritoneal cavity, which often causes painful menstruation and/or infertility.

Family—The people who mean well but can drive you a little nutty when you're fertility challenged.

Fertility Fish—A strange looking object meant to bring you good luck. Ours was probably mad at us for knocking it off the nightstand, so it may have held a grudge.

Fibroid Embolization—A non-surgical means of injecting arteries that supply blood to the fibroids with embolic agents to block the tumor's blood supply. A relatively new way of tackling fibroids, and therefore not recommended for women who are still trying to conceive.

Follicle—The place in the ovary where a woman's egg grows and develops each month. During ovulation, the follicle releases the egg into the fallopian tube.

Follicle Stimulating Hormone (FSH)—A hormone from the pituitary gland that stimulates ovarian follicles to grow.

Genetic Testing—A blood test for both partners to determine if there is a genetic defect causing infertility.

Gonadotropin—A hormone used during ovulation induction to encourage follicular and egg development.

Gonal F (Follitropin alfa, r-FSH)—A synthetic version of human follicle stimulating hormone indicated for women undergoing ovulation induction treatment and in assisted reproductive technology such as in vitro fertilization.

Human Chorionic Gonadotropin (hCG)—In early pregnancy, this hormone helps to maintain progesterone levels; it also used to trigger ovulation.

Hysteroscopy—An inspection of the uterine cavity with an endoscope via the cervix.

Hysterectomy—The partial or total removal of the uterus, ovaries and/or fallopian tubes.

Hysterosalpingo Contrast Sonography (HyCoSy)—An outpatient ultrasound procedure used to assess the condition of the fallopian tubes, as well as detect abnormalities of the uterus and endometrium using a non-iodine contrast agent.

Hysterosalpingogram (HSG Test)—An X-ray examination using a special dye injected into the uterus to observe the uterus and fallopian tubes.

Implantation—After fertilization, the egg embeds into the uterine lining where it starts to develop as an embryo.

In Vitro Fertilization (IVF)—Meaning "in glass," this assisted reproductive technology involves ovulation induction, extraction of the egg from the ovary, and combining the egg with the sperm outside of the female's body for fertilization.

Infertility—The inability to get pregnant or carry a pregnancy to term when trying to conceive.

Injectables—Fertility medications (usually ovulation induction medications) that are injected.

Intrauterine Insemination (IUI)—Sperm are collected and washed to prepare for insemination directly into a woman's uterus with a catheter and syringe.

Laparoscope—A telescopic instrument that is inserted into a small incision in the abdomen, for viewing of the pelvis, ovaries, uterus and fallopian tubes.

Laparoscopy—The direct visualization of the ovaries, outside of tubes and uterus via a laparoscope.

Lupron—Sometimes used in assisted reproduction cycles to suppress the pituitary gland—the gland responsible for triggering ovulation—along with briefly stimulating the pituitary to increase the pituitary hormones LH and FSH.

Luteinizing Hormone (LH)—A hormone that stimulates the ovary to release an egg during ovulation.

Luteal Phase—After ovulation, the final phase of the menstrual cycle that ends with pregnancy or menses. This phase often lasts between 12-14 days.

Luteal Phase Defect or Deficiency (LPD)—In a short luteal phase, the uterus will not be able to sustain a pregnancy due to abnormal hormone levels. LPD may cause recurrent miscarriages.

Miscarriage—Spontaneous loss of the embryo or fetus from the uterus before the 20th week of pregnancy. Occurs in about 20% of all pregnancies.

Misoprostol (Cytotec)—Used in combination with mifepristone to speed up the miscarriage process (complete or incomplete) and reduce the need for uterine curettage.

Ovarian Cyst—A fluid-filled sac in the ovary.

Ovidrel—A human chorionic gonadotropin injectable drug used to cause ovulation and treat infertility.

Ovulation—When the ovary releases a mature egg in the middle of the menstrual cycle, often around day 14. This is the most fertile time of a woman's cycle.

Ovulation Disorder—Infrequent or absent ovulation (anovulation), which results in infrequent periods or no periods at all.

Ovulation Predictor Kit/Ovulation Test)—Measures the luteinizing hormone (LH) in the urine, which spikes 24-48 hours prior to ovulation.

Pregnancy Test (including hCG, Estradiol, Progesterone Counts)—Either in urine or blood test form, pregnancy tests are designed to measure the amount of human chorionic gonadotropin, the hormone produced after a fertilized egg attaches to the uterus.

Premature Ovarian Failure (POF)—A syndrome associated with high levels of gonadotropins and low levels of estrogen, often causing menstruation to end before age 40.

Progesterone—The hormone that prepares the uterus for pregnancy after ovulation.

Progesterone Shots/Supplements—Typically given in the first trimester to help sustain pregnancy. There may not be enough progesterone made by the ovary during an IVF cycle, and so more progesterone is routinely given.

Progesterone Test—A blood test taken after ovulation to test the level of progesterone, necessary for implantation.

Semen Analysis—Examination of semen under a microscope to assess sperm count, movement (motility), and the size and shape of the sperm. See Appendix C for more details.

Sonogram (Ultrasound)—High-frequency sound waves used to monitor pregnancy and observe images of internal body parts.

"The Voice"—The "nearly whispered, dripping with concern, are you sure you aren't going postal" voice family often uses when they are worried about you.

"Those People"—The women who complain when it takes them more than a month to get pregnant!

Ultrasound—High-frequency sound waves used to monitor pregnancy and observe images of internal body parts (also called a sonogram).

Ultrasound-Guided Embryo Transfer/Sono-Guided Embryo Transfer—Embryos are transferred into the uterus guided by ultrasound. Research shows this can increase implantation and pregnancy rates.

Uterine Fibroid—A benign (non-cancerous) tumor made of muscle cells and other tissues that develop in the uterus or uterine lining. Also called myomas, firomyomas or leiomyomas. See Appendix B for more information on fibroids.

Unexplained Infertility—When no reason or cause can be found for a couple's infertility problems.

Vaginal Ultrasound—Placing a probe into the vagina and using sound waves to view the follicles, ovaries, eggs, fetus and other internal organs.

APPENDIX B
MORE ABOUT FIBROIDS

Fibroid tumors are solid masses made of fibrous tissue (hence the name) typically found in the uterus. They may grow as a single nodule or in a cluster and they vary greatly in size—from microscopic to large grapefruits. (Can you imagine a ball of flesh the size of a grapefruit growing in your uterus? Ouch!) They are generally benign (non-cancerous) and they often cause no symptoms, though 25% of the time they do cause side effects such as abnormal bleeding, painful menstrual cycles, backaches, and if the tumor is large enough, a swollen abdomen and bladder issues (it's easy to imagine something the size of a grapefruit doing that).

Fibroid tumors are common in women in their 30s and 40s—the most common being intramural fibroids, located inside the wall of the uterus. Subserosal fibroids develop outside of the uterus and usually produce the least symptoms. Submucosal fibroids are the least desirable of the three (not that having fleshy grapefruit grow anywhere in your uterus is at all desirable). Found within the uterine lining and sometimes protruding into the uterine cavity, they are the most difficult to remove.

Feel like you're back in science class yet?

The cause of uterine fibroids is unknown, but many believe there is a link to estrogen, as they do not develop before menstruation and they tend to shrink or disappear with the onset of menopause. The use of birth control pills and estrogen replacement therapy often speeds the growth of fibroids. They are the "Miracle Grow" for fibroids.

Most fibroids do not require treatment, but when it's determined that a fibroid should be removed, the only permanent options are surgical in nature. At a high level, the four main options are a laparoscopy, myomectomy, hysterectomy or fibroid embolization.

For women who want to bear children, a hysterectomy, or removal of the uterus, is not an option (unless you pull off the whole immaculate conception thing). And while fibroid embolization, where the flow of blood to the tumor is cut off by injecting tiny particles into the artery feeding it, is the least invasive procedure of the four, there are currently not enough studies on future fertility impact to warrant trying that route. So much for the easy (or at least "easier") route.

Most women who need to remove a fibroid start with a laparoscopy. It is a minor surgery performed under general anesthesia in an outpatient setting. A laparoscope (picture a miniature telescope with a fiber optic light at the end about the diameter of a fountain pen and twice as long) is inserted through a tiny incision in the abdomen. Two other small incisions at the pubic hairline are made for surgical tools. The fibroid can only be removed during a laparoscopy if a large portion of the tumor is located inside the uterine cavity, but the exact location is often unknown until the doctor begins the procedure. An exploratory laparoscopy may be necessary anyway to diagnose and treat endometriosis (the presence of endometrial tissue in locations outside the uterine cavity), which can be a cause of fertility problems.

If you're out of luck removing the fibroid via laparoscopy, the next step is a myomectomy, which requires a larger incision (three inches versus three centimeters) and longer recovery time (two to six weeks versus two days).

APPENDIX C
SEMEN ANALYSIS

A fresh semen sample, not more than half an hour old, after sexual abstinence for 2 days, is checked for the following characteristics:

Volume—A measure of how much semen is present. Normal volume of ejaculate in healthy men is about 2 to 6 ml.

Count—A count of the number of sperm present per milliliter of semen. The average sperm count in healthy men is 20-40 million sperm per ml.

Morphology—A measure of the percentage of sperm that have a normal shape. A good sperm should have a regular oval head with a connecting mid-piece and a long straight tail. A normal sample should have at least 15% of sperm with a normal shape.

Motility—A measure of the percentage of sperm that can move forward. A normal result is at least 20% of the sperm showing progressive movement in a forward direction.

pH—A measure of the acidity or alkalinity of the semen. Normal semen is alkaline, protecting the sperm from the acidity of the vaginal fluid.

Liquefaction Time/Viscosity—A measure of the time it takes the semen to liquefy. A liquefaction time within 60 minutes is within normal range.

Fructose Level—A measure of the amount of sugar in the semen (fructose provides energy for the sperm). Its absence suggests a block in the male reproductive tract.

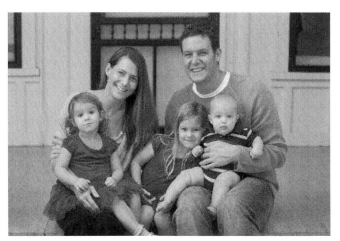

Michelle, Chris, Sydney, Sabrina & Luke

Proof

Made in the USA
Charleston, SC
18 June 2014